MEETING THE CHALLENGE OF ARTHRITIS

Also by Michael Brant Shermer:

Cycling: Endurance and Speed

Psychling: On Mental and Physical Fitness

The RAAM Book

Sport Cycling

Teach Your Child Science

The Woman Cyclist (with Elaine Mariolle)

MEETING THE CHALLENGE OF ARTHRITIS

A Motivational Program to Help You Live a Better Life

George Yates
Michael Brant Shermer

LOWELL HOUSE
Los Angeles
CONTEMPORARY BOOKS
Chicago

Library of Congress Cataloging in Publication Data

Yates, George.
    Meeting the challenge of arthritis: a motiva-
tional program to help you live a better life /
George Yates and Michael Shermer.
        p.   cm.
    Includes bibliographical references and index.
    ISBN 0–929923–28–6
    1. Arthritis—Popular works. 2. Arthritis—
Patients—Rehabilitation. 3. Arthritis—
Psychological aspects. I. Shermer, Michael. II.
Title.
RC933.Y37 1990   90–43098
616.7 ' 22—dc20   CIP

    LOWELL HOUSE
    1875 Century Park East, Suite 220
    Los Angeles, CA 90067

Publisher: JACK ARTENSTEIN

Vice-President/Editor-in-Chief: JANICE GALLAGHER

Marketing Manager: ELIZABETH WOOD

Design: MIKE YAZZOLINO

Manufactured in the United States of America

10   9   8   7   6   5   4   3   2   1

"Out of the night that covers me,
Black as the Pit from pole to pole,
I thank whatever gods may be
For my unconquerable soul.
It matters not how strait the gate,
How charged with punishments the scroll,
I am the master of my fate;
I am the captain of my soul."

WILLIAM ERNEST HENLEY, *Invictus*

I wish to dedicate this book to a number of individuals who saw me through the ordeals and triumphs of dealing with arthritis:

My Parents
for their care and guidance from beginning to end and for believing in my goals and aspirations.

Dr. John Curd
for helping me overcome both the physical and mental barriers that confronted me and for telling me I could do it.

Michael Shermer
for helping me over that first "hill" and who shared the dream that I would once again reach the top of the mountain.

Theresa
whose undying devotion gave me the courage to keep going even on the days when the pain stripped me of my confidence.

Acknowledgments

I would like to acknowledge Ross Laboratories and Exceed Sports Nutritionals for their support, as well as Neo-Life Company of America for supplying me with nutritional products. I would like to thank our editor, Janice Gallagher, who was invaluable in shaping this book into a highly readable and comprehensible text without any sacrifice of quality and accuracy. Thanks also to Derek Gallagher and Patti Cohen who were instrumental in producing a book that alleviated the fears all authors have of how the final product will look, and to Jack Artenstein for the opportunity to write this book.

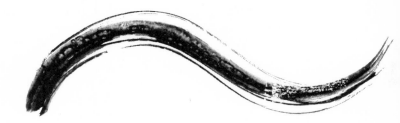

Contents

The Physical Challenge

"There are no great men, only great challenges that ordinary men are forced by circumstances to meet."

—ADMIRAL WILLIAM F. HALSEY

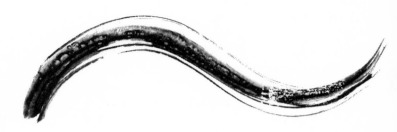

The first topic that must be addressed in any book on arthritis is the disease itself. What is arthritis and what can you do about it? But there is more to this disease than just the physical aspects. There is a mental side as well. *Meeting the Challenge of Arthritis* integrates both physical and mental challenges. The second half of the book primarily focuses on the psychological components involved in the disease, from beginning to end; from first realizing you have the disease to reaching a state of happiness and satisfaction in learning to live with it—that is, learning to be a participant again. Therefore part 2 contains the main principles of the *mental challenge* concept.

But we must begin at the beginning, the *physical challenge*. Part 1 covers a personal observation by Michael Shermer on my comeback from debilitating arthritis and how my motivational program for rehabilitation can help you live a better life (chapter 1); my personal account of how this book came to be written and for whom it was written (chapter 2); a general discussion of what arthritis is and what you can do about it from a medical point of view (chapter 3); the latest on arthritis and exercise and why old ideas about arthritis are giving way to new concepts that encourage an active approach to the disease (chapter 4); and a review of the controversial subject of arthritis and nutrition, looked at from both my personal experiences and experiments, and what the scientific evidence tells us (chapter 5).

OPTIMIZING THE ARTHRITIS CHALLENGE

These introductory chapters are important to establish the ground rules of the *physical challenge,* in order to then learn the rules to meet the *mental challenge.* Since so little has been written on the mental side of arthritis, and everyone who has the disease deals with it in his or her own unique way, then both authors and readers are breaking new ground together. In this second part, you'll also be hearing from others who have met the challenge of arthritis successfully.

Breaking new ground, of course, means that we can't guarantee results. The point of this book, however, is not to offer guarantees of arthritis relief or cure, but to *optimize* your chances for dealing with arthritis in a fulfilling manner.

One of the motivations for me to write this book was that when I first got out of the hospital and was in so much pain I was very open to any and all suggestions to get some relief. I headed straight for a health food bookstore and found a number of books whose titles all had the words *arthritis relief* in them. I bought these books, read them, and proceeded to drain my bank account purchasing all sorts of special foods, vitamins, minerals, and supplements, all of which were supposed to relieve my arthritis pain, and none of which did. This angered me, but in the process I kept track of all the different claims, did numerous experiments on myself, and eventually filtered out the sense from the nonsense and arrived at what I think is a reasonable program for *optimizing* the arthritis challenge. This book is the result of this filtering process.

1

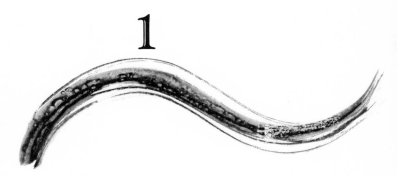

A Man to Match My Mountain
A Personal Observation
by Michael Shermer

"Here is a hero who did nothing but shake the tree when the fruit was ripe. Do you think that was a small thing to do? Well, just look at the tree he shook."

—FRIEDRICH NIETZSCHE
HUMAN ALL-TOO-HUMAN

One morning in April 1984 my coauthor George Yates awoke to a nightmare that surpassed any he had ever had while asleep—he was wracked with arthritic pain so debilitating that he couldn't get out of bed. Sound familiar? If you're reading this book it probably does. But the story gets worse. George didn't know he had arthritis. In fact, only a few short months before he had swum 2.4 miles in the open ocean, cycled 112 miles in 100-degree heat, and run a 26-mile marathon—all in one day at the Ironman Triathlon! And now he couldn't even get out of bed, and I mean he *literally* could not get out of bed—he simply could not move a muscle.

In chapter 2 George will tell the story of what happened to him in his own words—how he went from professional athlete to bedridden arthritic, to professional athlete once again. This is a story for all of us who at some time must struggle with adversity. As George grappled to comprehend what was happening to him, and as I stood by, unable to offer anything more than sympathy and support, the outline of this book took shape. George once again competes in the Ironman, but the road from there to here—from virtual paralysis to near-complete recovery—was long, rocky, and circuitous.

A STORY WITH A MESSAGE

This book is not about one man's journey; rather, it is about what George learned along the way—what dead-ends he encountered and what forks in the road he faced, and how he made critical decisions that led to a state of relative health and happiness as he continues to live with arthritis. Those lessons have been developed into a motivational program to help you live a better life and to help you become a participant again, as you daily meet the challenges of arthritis.

I've known George for 10 years, and while he and I are the best of friends, he has become something bigger than that to me—a hero of sorts, though friends are not usually heroes, nor heroes friends. Joseph Campbell once remarked: "A hero is someone who has given his or her life to something bigger than oneself." George has unwittingly had to face a challenge bigger than himself—arthritis—and he has given his life to understanding it, overcoming it, and helping others to do the same. This is what I mean in calling George a hero.

A Hero's Adventure

When I first met George Yates in 1980 he had been a national-class bicycle road racer for nearly 10 years. George was making the transition to the triathlon movement just when the Hawaiian Ironman competition was gaining fame in *Sports Illustrated* and on ABC's "Wide World of Sports." In triathlons George found his own best destiny, and quickly moved up the ranks into the top 10. In the Ironman, if you finish in the top 50 you are considered a phenomenal athlete, in the top 25 you're one of the best, and in the top 10 you're almost deified. George finished seventh in 1982, and set his sights on winning the race in 1983.

The year 1983 was a good training year for both George and me. He was preparing for the Ironman, while I was getting ready for the 3,000-mile nonstop Race Across America (RAAM). We rode the 23-mile, 6,000-foot climb from my house to the top of Mt. Wilson at least once a week. It was George who kept me motivated. George was a training fanatic. He never missed a beat. Up at six for a couple of thousand yards of swimming, then a long hard ride.

At the end of one of these training rides I was dead-tired. The only running I was up for was a short run from the shower to the kitchen. George, on the other hand, usually followed these arduous training rides with a 10- to 15-mile run! Rested and recovered from my stint at the trough, I'd meet George, following his run, at the weight room and watch in awe as he'd push himself through a rigorous program of stretching and weights to increase his flexibility and strength.

What was so inspiring about George was not just the quantity of his exercise, which was considerable, or even the quality of exercise, which was of the highest order, but his consistency from day to day. George used to say to me that if he missed a day it was "back to square one." It is a philosophy that paid off in results—George had many an impressive victory.

Toward the end of that 1983 training season I noticed George slowing down a bit and complaining of always being tired and sore. His joints were stiff, and he seemed to be getting injured a lot. I thought perhaps this was due to overtraining, and recommended he slow down a bit and even take a day off. Reluctantly he did, but it didn't seem to help. He went to the Ironman, and instead of winning, or finishing in the top 10, or top 25, he finished 48th. This, of course, would be outstanding to most of the 1,500 entrants, but not to someone who had grown accustomed to racing in the top 10.

After the Ironman I didn't see or speak to George for a few months, and I wondered what had happened to him in the Ironman. He had told me that he was tired and that he had slightly injured himself before the race, but it didn't make sense—George should have easily finished at least in the top 20. The following spring I got a phone call from George that answered all my questions and left me in a state of shock. George was phoning from the Scripps Clinic in San Diego and suddenly the full horror of what had transpired over that period of time came to light. George had been stricken with arthritis, diagnosed as acute ankylosing spondylitis—a spinal arthritis for which there is no cure. During the entire 1983 season, and on all those training rides, George was carrying that virus around inside him. By the Ironman it had really begin to spread. Within a few months following the Ironman he was no longer able to train. Then on that fateful morning in April, George was in so much pain, in every joint of his body, that he couldn't even get out of bed. He couldn't even reach the phone.

Conquering the Mountain

In the next chapter George will fill in the details of his disease and recovery program. But let me tell just one story that I think symbolizes George's indefatigable spirit—his drive to never give up. George called me one day, fairly early on in his rehabilitation program, to ask me if I would assist him in his first bike ride. This seemed inconceivable to me because just the month before we had gone to lunch together, and the walk from the parking lot to the restaurant left an imprint on my mind that will never be erased. *It took us a full 10 minutes just to cross the street!* George could barely lift his leg up the curb onto the sidewalk. How in the world could he expect to ride a bike? I worried about my friend's frame of mind, but figured he knew his body better than anyone else.

We drove up to the Rose Bowl in Pasadena, which has a flat, 3.2-mile road course surrounding it. But for George, the tiniest of bumps might as well have been mountains. But in his inimitable fashion he refused a push until he was moving so slowly that he was nearly falling over.

We did three very slow laps in all and proclaimed it a victory, but it was still a long way from Mt. Wilson, where we used to ride. Ironically, from a certain vantage point at the Rose Bowl, you can see the towers and observatory buildings atop Mt. Wilson. After those three laps George pointed up there and said, "Someday, Shermer, we're going back." I couldn't in my wildest imagination picture that happening again. I was certainly impressed—amazed really—that George was able to ride three laps. I was very proud of his courage to get out there and even attempt that feat. But Mt. Wilson? Never. I was wrong. Within three months George and I rode all the way up to the top of that mountain.

If you took a fictional script to a film producer and told him you had this story about an ex-triathlete who was totally paralyzed by arthritis, and that in less than two years this same arthritic would be hammering out of the saddle, pounding away on the pedals, for 23 miles on an eight percent graded mountain road to the top of an astronomical observatory, and then later that year he would go back to the Ironman and finish the race, he'd probably say, "Get outta here, no one will believe it!" George Yates matched and conquered that mountain, and has finished every Ironman triathlon since, proving that the truth is often stranger and more wonderful than fiction.

THE PURPOSE OF THIS BOOK

This book, then, on one level, is a statement of hope for all told they have arthritis. The book is a motivational program designed around a statement George made to the more than 37 million arthritis victims in the United States in *Reader's Digest* last year (March 1989), and symbolizes what *meeting the challenge of arthritis* means: "I want all of them to know they don't have to accept this disease passively—that they should take their problems by the scruff of the neck and *deal* with them. The way to make positive things happen is to find the right help, set realistic goals, and do what it takes to meet them. Don't let anything ruin the only life you have to live."

George and I feel we have struck a chord in this motivational program that will resonate the power of motivation in everyone who wants to try. Since the *Reader's Digest* article was published, George has received many letters from arthritis sufferers all over the country, acknowledging his frustration with the medical community in its inability to deal with the mental challenge of arthritis. For example, we believe this letter from Ms. Joanna Innatowicz from El Cajon, California is symbolic of a large portion of the millions of arthritis sufferers in this country who would like to take their arthritis by the scruff of the neck, but have never been encouraged to do so:

December 11, 1989

Dear Mr. Yates:

I read your story in the *Reader's Digest* with more than just a passing interest. I am not a triathlete (not even close) nor have I been diagnosed with ankylosing spondylitis or Reiter's syndrome (merely intermittent anthralgias and a recurring bone spur which pinches a spinal nerve in my cervical area and sends shooting pains down my arm). What I have always been is a physically active individual and I resent the incapacity that pain has imposed on me. But what additionally angers me is the attitude of the medical establishment in that all they can offer me is some different anti-inflammatory agent, not a regimen of exercise that might take me out of a pain-induced inactivity.

What intrigued me in the article was a statement of your goal—to get the message across to the 37 million arthritis sufferers, to "find the right help, set realistic goals, and do what it takes to meet them." I am not involved in the sports arena; my goals are more modest—to involve myself in an organized program that would let me keep my body in the best possible shape consistent with a modest investment of time due to full-time job commitments. The key is: *to find the right help.* Can you advise whom I could contact to obtain this type of advice and not just a disinterested shrug?

Sincerely,
Joanna Innatowicz

In two short paragraphs Ms. Innatowicz has summarized the problem, the solution, and to whom this book applies. Our motivational program is directed to anyone who is ready to meet the challenge of arthritis by taking the problem by the "scruff of the neck." Our program is basically designed around the three themes of finding the right help, setting realistic goals, and doing what it takes to meet them. The first half of the book, the physical challenge, covers the basics of arthritis: what it is, what you can do about it, and where to find the right help.

The second half of the book, the mental challenge, is what we believe sets our book apart from all others in this field. It addresses the complaints of so many arthritis sufferers—summarized in Ms. Innatowicz's letter—that the medical establishment has little to offer other than physical forms of intervention, such as anti-inflammatory agents. We believe there are mental forms of intervention as well, and it is these we address in part 2 of the book: turning your arthritis into a new challenge; designing goals to meet that new challenge, learning how to achieve those goals, and how to deal with failure when it comes. We then try to integrate the physical and mental challenge into a program that includes healthy nutrition, exercise, and a balanced lifestyle to help you lead a better life.

For Family and Friends of Arthritis Sufferers

We also want to note that this book is applicable to and important for friends and family members of arthritis sufferers to read. One of the key points in the motivational program is to build around yourself a powerful support structure that focuses on close friends and family members. These are the people you deal with daily, the individuals who have seen you at your worst, and can now help you become your best. In this sense meeting the challenge of arthritis is a team program. You are the quarterback, calling the plays and taking responsibility for the outcome of the game, but your family and friends are the running backs, receivers, and linemen who will make it possible for you to score the big play.

The significance of that support structure will become more important as the motivational program is developed in the second half of the book. Suffice it to say that when you design the program, you should do so not only with family and friends in mind, but they can help you with the design itself. This is what George did when he called me and others to help him with his rehabilitation. He surrounded himself with positive people who would encourage him to keep pushing and not give up.

A Program for Everyone

When we began work on this book I worried that many readers might think the program would not apply to them because of George's background as a professional athlete. But letters in response to the *Reader's Digest* article have convinced me that while very few are interested in doing *specifically* what George did—the Ironman—virtually everyone is interested in doing *generally* what George did—become a participant in life again. The Ironman in particular, and sports in general, are just an analogy for the successful life process of setting and achieving goals in order to lead a more fulfilling life. The specifics are not important. It's the general principles that count. This book is about those principles and how you can apply them to the specifics of *your* life.

For me, George personifies the hero in all of us. By Campbell's definition, all arthritis sufferers can be heroes by meeting the challenge of arthritis head-on. *What* George did is not as important as *how* he did it. Everyone is affected by arthritis in a different way, and there are so many types that no one program of *what* to do can meet the needs of everyone. So our program tells you *how* to meet the challenge of arthritis—both physically and mentally.

TOUCHING OTHERS' LIVES

There is, I believe, another message in this book, a message that runs deeper but can be found in everyone who has ever had to overcome adversity or take up a challenge. It is a statement of the power of the individual to make a difference, in his own life and in the life of others. Every one of us is connected to others through a myriad of linkages: the family members we live with or see regularly, the people with whom we work, those we meet occasionally, good friends and casual friends, and all those people who have relationships or interact with the people we know. Everything that any one of us does may affect innumerable others in countless indirect and probably unknown ways. Anything you do may affect another human being, which may alter someone else's actions, which affects still another event, which influences yet another person, and so on in a cascading series of contingent connections.

Perhaps an example would make my point clear. In 1979 I was a recent graduate in psychology, unable to find work teaching. Since I could write, I applied for a job with a bicycle magazine, though I had no particular interest in cycling. Steve Ready, the editor, hired me because I could write and at least had an interest in sports. The first day on the job Steve sent me to a press conference about John Marino, who had just ridden across America in 13 days. I was fascinated, we became friends, and I bought a bike the next day. Steve encouraged me to enter a race one week later. I did and enjoyed the event, so he and I began a series of rides and races every weekend. The longer the ride, the better I did. Inspired by John and encouraged by Steve, I did a 100-mile ride, then a 200-mile ride. Then I rode from Seattle to San Diego to raise money for charity to help my girlfriend who had recently been partially paralyzed in an automobile accident. This ride turned into an annual record attempt, which in 1982 brought me an invitation into the first Race Across America against John Marino and two other men. This also became an annual event, the training for which I did much of the time with a professional triathlete named George Yates whom I met when working for the bike magazine! So through a long series of connections I have come to write this book with George because in 1979 Steve Ready sent me on a news assignment. This is what I mean by contingent connections. There is simply no way of knowing how one thing might lead to another, and by whom you might be inspired, or whom you might inspire, to take up challenges.

This means that everything which you and I do counts. Thinking about these connections has made me cognizant of the importance of every one of our actions. What we do and say matters, and in this truth lies what I believe to be the loftier message of this book and why I agreed to coauthor it with George.

The main body of our work is for you the reader—a new manifesto of self-improvement in overcoming the seemingly crippling effects of disease. But there is something deeper, something that goes beyond the aggrandizement of self. That something is within, but really at the bedrock of George's story—touching other's lives by way of example. For me, George is a stunning model of the very principles outlined in this book: understanding the problem, setting and achieving goals to overcome the problem, and dealing with failure. The success George has achieved was done by his own design— George was truly the master of his fate. Such "come-from-behind" stories touch me deeply, but there is something yet to be discussed.

While this book is for you the reader, a secondary motive is for you the reader to become a shining example for still others. Every one of you has the opportunity to do what George has done. By this I do not mean the Ironman Triathlon or any other specific physical feat. But like George, you have the opportunity to turn your ordeal into a conquest; to convert this tribulation into a triumph—if not exclusively for yourself, then by example, for others.

As I write this chapter the day after Christmas (1989), I am reminded of that holiday classic movie presentation which I watched last night—Frank Capra's *It's a Wonderful Life*, starring Jimmy Stewart. Stewart plays George Bailey, a small-town building and loan proprietor who, after decades of hard, honest work feels his life has been a failure because he sees nothing of the results of his efforts. Some of his friends have left town to make more money. Others have gone to see the world. His own brother is a decorated war hero. But George has done seemingly little. His life seems stalled and stagnant, and when financial and familial pressures finally build beyond control on Christmas Eve, George exclaims that he wishes he were never born and then decides to take his life. Fortunately he is interrupted by his guardian angel who grants him his wish and shows him what his little town of Bedford Falls would have been like without him.

Suddenly things are not what they used to be, and the changes are mostly slanted toward the negative. The people George helped financially are instead poor and wretched, the buildings he constructed are nonexistent, his wife is a lonely spinster, his children unborn, and the town is renamed "Pottersville," after the greedy banker whose miserly ways prevented those George had helped from ever owning their own homes. His brother, whom George saved in childhood, is not there to save other lives in a specific battle of World War Two, with the contingent consequences that the lives the brother saved are now also gone. As the guardian angel guides George through his now unfamiliar surroundings, he is dismayed and shocked. He never realized just how many people were dependent upon his seemingly routine existence. "Strange, isn't it?," queries the angel to George at the appropriate moment of enlightenment. "Each man's life touches so many other lives, and when he isn't around he leaves an awful hole, doesn't he?"

In this sense, then, we are all individuals of power and importance. While no one desires a crippling disease, it does provide at least one important opportunity—the chance to touch others' lives by way of example. You are, in this sense then, at a crossroads, of sorts—a vista point from where you are looking down two roads—one of optimism and hope, the other of despair and gloom. This book is really one long argument for choosing the path of the former—the path that both George Bailey and George Yates chose. But whichever you decide, remember that whether you like it or not, whether you know it or not, the path you choose may affect uncounted others in multitudinous ways.

In my favorite example of this contingent nature of change, "The Road not Taken," Robert Frost reminds us that once we start down a chosen path there is no turning back. As we move down the road, we alter the road irrevocably ("way leads on to way"). Decisions are final and everlasting, and each and every one of us can cause change, even if it is not apparent. We all touch so many other lives that each fork in the road becomes one more chance to make a difference:

Two roads diverged in a yellow wood,
and sorry I could not travel both
and be one traveler, long I stood
and looked down one as far as I could
to where it bent in the undergrowth;

Then took the other, as just as fair,
and having perhaps the better claim,
because it was grassy and wanted wear;
Though as for that the passing there
had worn them really about the same.

And both that morning equally lay
in leaves no step had trodden black.
Oh, I kept the first for another day!
Yet knowing how way leads on to way,
I doubted if I should ever come back.

I shall be telling this with a sigh
somewhere ages and ages hence:
Two roads diverged in a wood, and I—
I took the one less traveled by,
and that has made all the difference.

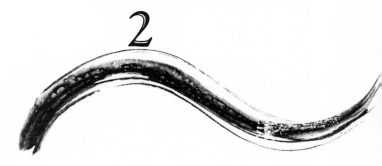

Ordeal and Triumph
A First-Person Account
by George Yates

"Never stop being ambitious. You have but one life, live it to the fullest glory and be willing to pay any price."

—General George S. Patton

When Michael Shermer and I decided to collaborate on this book, he insisted that I tell my own story. The reason, he argued, was that no one with arthritis would believe such results as I have had are possible, unless they could see that someone with arthritis had actually applied my principles successfully.

Well, I did, but I want to note that there is nothing in this book that claims I have any "secret" formula for success. I don't have a "magic" cure, nor do I tell you how to master some sort of "psychic" power to overcome your arthritis. There is nothing special about my arthritis, or how I dealt with it, that precludes your doing the same. One thing I learned about this disease is that there is no magic bullet.

The principles in this book are about as basic as they come, but as I discovered, when you are completely immobilized with pain, you need the basics, and nothing more. What sort of basics? Just fundamentals of goal setting and achievement, expanding your limitations, and dealing with failure. Integrating these principles, which I will discuss in the second half of the book, with the physical challenge of arthritis, can lead to a better life. It did for me. So, in a nutshell, this is what happened to me and how I applied these fundamental principles of the mental challenge to my arthritic condition.

OMINOUS WARNINGS

In the summer of 1983 I was 28 years old, a full-time professional triathlete, and in the best shape of my life. A triathlon is an event combining swimming, cycling, and running, ranging anywhere from "sprint" length triathlons to the Ironman Triathlon in Hawaii: a 2.4-mile swim, a 112-mile bike race, and a 26.2-mile marathon run. What I didn't know was that I was carrying in my body the seeds of rheumatoid arthritis. In September of that year, right after I finished the World Triathlon Championships in Nice, France, I began to feel something was wrong with my body. From France I went to Hawaii to prepare for the Ironman Triathlon, which was in October, and while I was training I found myself getting stiffer and sorer by the day. Well, I figured this was probably normal, since the Nice Triathlon was a long, hard race, and my training in Hawaii was unusually grueling. But when I awoke one morning and my back was painfully tight, I knew something was amiss. I couldn't even move my lower back—it was completely locked up. I remember it took me about 20 minutes of stretching just to get my back loosened up enough in order to walk normally. My body felt like a cold motor that needed a long warm-up just to get started.

I did the Ironman, and my results told me that something was wrong. The year before I had finished seventh, and this year I trained almost twice as hard, so I figured I'd be in the top five or maybe even win the race. Instead I finished in 48th place! I felt like someone had a rope tied around my waist and was pulling me back.

Then in January 1984 I went back to Hawaii for a triathlon called Kuaii Loves You. The day before the race I was running from the road through the parking lot to my room and I stumbled on a concrete parking block. I went down hard on the ground and threw my back out. I spent the rest of the day in bed in excruciating pain and competed in the race the next day, but in misery.

After that injury, my symptoms got progressively worse. I was beginning to experience pain in my arms and shoulders, feet, ankles, and knees. I kept hoping it was because of the new training season, or that I hadn't fully recovered from the Ironman. But week by week I was getting worse. It was so subtle that if I had not been working out a lot and this had happened I would have known something was definitely wrong. But because athletes do get sore from training, I kept hoping it was nothing abnormal. I was wrong.

The "Worst Possible" Scenario

My complete physical breakdown came on April 17, 1984. Within a day and a half I went from not feeling too well to being totally immobilized in bed. I'll never forget that week as long as I live. The Sunday before I was in a 75-mile bike race from Santa Ana College to the Scripps Clinic in La Jolla, California. I remember standing there at the finish line looking at Scripps and thinking to myself that I had always heard of this famous place but had never seen it. Little did I know that within a month I would be rolled in there by wheelchair as a patient.

Anyway, the race was on Sunday. On Monday morning I awoke and my whole body was locked up—pain in all my joints, especially my lower back. I managed to get out to my car and went to see a chiropractor/sports trainer friend of mine who told me to go home and rest and take it easy, and especially not to exercise.

Well, this was the worst thing I could have done! I didn't know it at the time, but it was my training that was preventing the total collapse of my body. So naively I went home to bed and hardly moved for five days. My friends came over to feed me and help out, but I didn't get better. The fact was, I got worse each day. I'd go to sleep and wake up with my left knee swollen to the size of a grapefruit. Then I'd fall back asleep and awaken to find my right ankle swollen like a softball! And so on. It got so I was afraid to fall asleep. Day by day, hour by hour, my joints were locking up so that by the fifth day I couldn't move at all. And nobody had a clue as to what was going on.

I kept thinking I should call a doctor, but then I also thought perhaps when I awoke I'd feel better. There was a certain amount of denial going on in this process, which I have since discovered that other people experience when they first get arthritis. You just don't want to believe there is something seriously wrong with your body.

Finally, on the fifth morning, I woke up with a fever, sweating and shaking, and desperate to go to the bathroom. It took me a full hour to move myself to the edge of the bed. I was so locked up with pain, inflammation, and stiffness that just trying to get out of bed was horrifying. Finally, I got myself to the edge of the bed, fell off, and grabbed the door. I started to fall so I clutched the door handle and tried to lift myself to my feet, but a hot poker-like pain shot through my back and I lost consciousness. When I came to I was lying on the bathroom floor with my feet under the toilet and my head under the sink. It's amazing I didn't smash my head against the sink. To make matters worse, I was incontinent. I hadn't gone to the bathroom for so long I just went there on the floor all over myself. I couldn't help it because I just couldn't move anymore. So there I was, this 28-year-old professional athlete lying in my own waste, feeling at one and the same time terror, anger, and utter helplessness.

Finally, after I had been lying there for a couple of hours, one of my buddies came over to check on me. When he looked in and didn't see me in the bed, he yelled out for me and I screamed for him to come into the bathroom. When he found me on the floor, he was shocked. I looked like hell.

From One Hell to Another

My buddy called the paramedics immediately and they came with the sirens blaring. My neighbors clustered around. Three or four paramedics came into the house and couldn't figure out what was wrong with me. They put a sheet over me and tried to move me onto a stretcher, but the pain of their even touching me was so excruciating that I was screaming bloody murder. Everything hurt—even my skin.

Finally they moved me in rapid bursts, during which I screamed in pain, until they finally got me onto the stretcher and into the ambulance. They drove me to Hoag Memorial Hospital, which was only about six miles away; but it took them an hour to make the journey. They couldn't drive at a normal speed because each bump and movement of the ambulance caused me to scream. So we traveled down the side of the road at five or six miles an hour.

The doctors at the emergency room couldn't figure out what was wrong, so they gave me all kinds of tests. No one even thought of arthritis. Finally, after about 45 minutes they announced that all tests were negative. They wanted to send me back home to get some rest! I couldn't believe it. I said no way. We argued about it for awhile until I had them call my chiropractor friend. When he got to the hospital he couldn't believe his eyes. He insisted the doctors admit me. Someone finally gave me a shot of Demerol and I lost consciousness. This was about 11:00 in the morning. I woke up at 9:30 that night.

When I awoke, the doctors started more tests. They stuck a huge needle into my hip and removed some fluid, which contained inflammatory pus. After analyzing it, the doctor told me I was being admitted to the hospital. What threw the doctors at first was my age and physique. Like me, they just never imagined a 28-year-old athlete having such severe arthritis.

LIFE WITHOUT HOPE?

I was at Hoag Memorial Hospital for two weeks, while the doctors were doing test after test and finding absolutely nothing. Meanwhile I was getting progressively worse. Finally they ran one last test—a test for a genetic marker for rheumatoid arthritis, which turned out positive. This was the first time that the word "arthritis" was even mentioned. I couldn't believe it. My image of an arthritis patient was someone much older, someone in physical decline. I just couldn't imagine it affecting a young person, especially someone like me.

The next day the doctor came in and told me that my case was extremely severe—worse than anything ever seen at Hoag in someone my age. He also told me there was absolutely no hope of my ever recovering from this condition and that I should resign myself to leading a highly medicated, sedentary lifestyle. Then he left. I was furious at the way this doctor had dealt with me after I had lost 40 pounds, developed bedsores, couldn't move, and was totally confused about my future. That was the last thing I needed to hear. But what really got me was that he didn't know anything about me as a person. He hadn't asked what I did for a living. He had no clue that I was a professional athlete. And he didn't know that I had inner strength to fight this thing.

So I checked out of the hospital immediately and went home, where I could at least be in a positive environment with my friends and family who would encourage me to get better. I called my mom and dad to come down and help me figure out what to do. I told my parents, "I want out of here. I don't buy this *no hope* prognosis." So they put me in a wheelchair and took me back to my house. I stayed there for a few days, until my mom remembered hearing about Scripps in La Jolla where they take unusual cases for research and treatment. Scripps is a leading research hospital where they are willing to try more experimental treatments and cutting-edge technology on patients.

The First Ray of Light

Three days later I checked into Scripps. The first doctor I met was John Curd, who was positive and encouraging. He began by experimenting with different drugs to see if any would have an effect. For days nothing happened, but Dr. Curd never became discouraged. He told me, "We'll do everything we can." Just hearing that gave me a boost. It was the first positive thing I had heard since my ordeal began. He kept trying different things until finally I started seeing just a little progress. What they found out was that drugs that were normally effective didn't work on me, and ones that shouldn't have worked seemed to help. That was the first lesson I learned—arthritis is a very individual disease. Everyone's body reacts slightly differently. So no doctor can ever tell you there is no hope, since no one can possibly know your body as well as you do.

Meanwhile, they were draining my knees and hips every day with a huge needle and sucking out a yellowish-looking fluid that was so thick it kept me from being able to bend my knees and move my legs. To this day I remember the doctor coming into my room with a needle the size of a carpet needle. The memory of that pain still haunts me to this day. But Dr. Curd was encouraging. I was feeling a little better and he kept urging me to try to move—even just a little.

What made Dr. Curd different from the other doctors was that he asked about *me*. He wanted to know what I did and who I was. He wanted to know what was going on in my mind. So I told him about the Ironman and that I was a professional athlete and had no intention of staying in bed. He then asked me what my goals were now that it was confirmed that I had arthritis. So I told him everything I was feeling, including the fact that I was determined to compete in the Ironman again. And instead of looking at me as if I were crazy, he told me he would do everything he could to help me realize my dream.

Then he took me to the staff psychologist to make sure that I was of "sound mind." I remember taking a series of psychological tests to assess my personality and my goals in life. The test results told him that I was, indeed, of a sound mind. So Dr. Curd informed me that the psychologist had given me the thumbs-up, and said who was he to think I couldn't make it all the way back? We laid out a plan of recovery and Dr. Curd let me know that he could only take me so far with the drug therapy and the rest would be up to me.

THE LONG ROAD BACK

After three weeks at Scripps, I was released and went back home to begin my rehabilitation. I called up a sports medicine specialist, Dr. Kenneth Forsythe, who said he would work with me to design a program. I told him my long-range goal was to compete in the Ironman Triathlon again in October of 1985. This was June 1984, so I had 16 months to prepare. This goal gave me something to shoot for; something to look down the road at when I was going through the monotony of rehab. As I was to discover, having a goal was pivotal to my recovery and has thus become an integral part of my motivational program for becoming a participant again.

I embarked upon my rehab by working out three to four days a week. Then I progressed to every day, always keeping in mind my ultimate goal of the Ironman. At first I couldn't even imagine running or cycling, because I could barely move my arms and legs. But slowly, day by day, I worked on my range of motion, my strength, and my endurance. This went on for a year. I went in with a walker and crutches and came out on my own. But don't think that it was one long steady rate of improvement. There were a lot of ups and downs. Sometimes I'd go for weeks without any improvement, then suddenly I'd get a jolt of strength and flexibiity. Then maybe I'd lose it for awhile, then get it back, and so on for months on end, until finally I was really able to get around on my own. It was a long process. I used thousands of ice packs over that period, icing my joints down after each workout.

The whole rehabilitation process was a step-by-step series of goals. From June through August 1984, I was just trying to get back my joint mobility and learn to walk without a walker or crutches. I remember driving up to Michael's house in Tustin, California to meet him at a restaurant. It was one of the first times that I walked somewhere without any support. It was a slow, painful process. It took us 10 minutes just to walk across the street. I finally made it to my table. I remember that being quite an accomplishment!

In September I started swimming every day. Swimming is good therapy because it's easy on the joints. The next big step after that was trying to ride a bike. Riding a bike is normally a smooth, nonstressful process—unless you fall! Crashing on my bike at this point would have been a complete disaster. But I was willing to take the risk. I met Michael at the Rose Bowl in Pasadena and we did a couple of laps around a reasonably flat 3.2-mile loop. But I remember this one little bump that I could barely get over and Michael was right there ready to catch me if I fell. After those laps I looked up and saw the communications towers atop Mt. Wilson, our old training ride that includes 6,000 feet and 23 miles of climbing from where we stood. I said, "Shermer, someday we're going to ride back up there again." It was kind of a long shot from where I stood (physically, that is), but I knew if I couldn't cimb that mountain, I would never be able to do the Ironman.

This period was a very emotional one for me. There was a lot at stake in nearly everything I tried, so I was always both apprehensive and excited. Apprehensive that should I fail I would have found my limit—and it would be too low to compete again. Excited, because every hurdle made me that much more confident in my strength, endurance, and mental stamina. Every extra lap in the pool, every additional trip around the Rose Bowl, made me stronger, both physically and mentally.

Then, between October 1984, when I first rode the bike, and March 1985, when I tried running, I worked on flexibility and strength. It is unbelievable how quickly bed rest causes you to lose muscle strength and bulk. In March I started jogging again to the point where I could almost run. My knees were still so sore that running was the biggest challenge. In May 1985 I entered a mini-triathlon just to see how I was doing compared to "regular" athletes. It was the triathlon at Bonelli Park in San Dimas and I finished 48th out of 500 people, so I did pretty well. I hurt like hell when it was over, but I knew that I wasn't completely unrealistic in my expectations of going back to Hawaii.

After that race I was really motivated! I started training like a madman—swimming, cycling, running, weights— every single day. With each day, week, and month I got stronger and stronger. By October 1985, when I returned to Hawaii, I was ready for the big test.

THE ULTIMATE CHALLENGE

Going back to Hawaii was really an emotional experience. I just couldn't believe I had come this far. I had regained most of the 40 pounds I had lost since I was first struck down, and now I was about to find out how much of my strength and endurance I had recovered. There were about 1,300 entrants. I was 75th out of the water after 2.4 miles of open-ocean swimming; and by the end of the 112-mile bike leg I was in 6th place! I knew then I had come back all the way. I knew, that is, until about 19 miles into the run. At that point I was starting to slow down and people passed me. By the 20th mile I was in 18th place.

Finally, my knees hurt so much and my joints were locking up, that I had to jog, and then finally walk. By the end, I could barely even move. The last mile or two I was in complete agony. Another 115 people passed me and I finished 134th overall. I guess it was just a little much for my body— but what a long way back from that day on my bathroom floor! I went there just hoping to finish and do the best I could do. I never dreamed I'd be in sixth place at the end of the bike leg and well into the run. This experience taught me one very important thing about arthritis: Most of the doctors and "authorities" in the field do not know what the real limitations are with this disease. They sell people short by not encouraging arthritis sufferers to reach for higher goals and dare mightier things. I'm sure there must be legal reasons for not pushing patients too far, but the arthritic person looks to these experts for encouragement to push onward, and they usually don't give it. But Dr. Curd and Dr. Forsythe gave me that one small ray of hope, and I took it and ran with it as far as I could.

BEYOND THE CHALLENGE

Athletics and the Ironman, for me, are the ultimate challenge. But the challenge goes far beyond just the physical.

There is the whole mental aspect as well, which integrates with the physical. But there is a challenge beyond both the physical and the mental. It is the challenge for life—having goals. For me, the Ironman is that yearly check on my health and fitness. I do it to keep that long-range goal out there so I have something to work toward each year. That is what life is all about—having goals and working toward improving yourself in whatever areas you consider important.

It isn't always one long road to success. In the 1986 Ironman, for example, my arthritis was really giving me problems and I had to walk the entire marathon. Imagine walking 26.2 miles. I finished a dismal 911th out of 1,039. But in 1987 I felt a lot better again, and finished 193rd out of 1,381 people. In 1988 I finished 330th out of 1,275 entrants. And so it goes, year after year. I'll keep doing the Ironman and other races because this is how I have chosen to live with my disease. I've still got arthritis. I still take the anti-inflammatory drug Feldene. I still wake up in the morning stiff and sore, but I get out there and work out every day. And overall, after six years of having arthritis, I can say that I feel stronger and healthier than ever, since being struck down in 1984.

This is what I mean about the challenge beyond the physical and mental aspects. Before getting arthritis, the Ironman was a great physical test, but it didn't mean what it does now. Now it is a constant reminder for me to keep pushing myself and to keep those goals out there in front of me. Every one of you has your own "Ironman"—that something special you want to do but are afraid you can't. Once you get over the fear and realize that it is the striving after the goal that counts, then you will know what I mean about moving beyond the challenge.

Having arthritis is a challenge for life. This is why I've gotten involved in the Arthritis Foundation. This is why I'm writing this book. I want to tell people not to accept everything that the authorities in the field tell them. While I respect the knowledge that the traditional medical community has, one thing it doesn't have is your knowledge of your own body. No one knows you like you do, and the only person who can put limitations on you is you. No doctor can tell you that you *absolutely* can or cannot do something. The only way to find out is to set a goal and try for it. *That's* how you discover your limitations. They aren't listed in a medical textbook.

Overall, I've come into the field of arthritis research at a crucial turning point, where medical doctors and physical therapists *are* recognizing the importance of exercise for the mobility of an arthritic body. In a way, I was sort of an unwitting test case. Not that I was the first. But I came along at a time when at least some doctors—and mine was one of them—thought that exercise was good for arthritis. Now doctors are much more likely to tell patients to go out and exercise to get the blood pumping and the joints limber. Lying in bed, not moving, is probably the worst thing many arthritics can do. But again I want to emphasize that only *you* know for sure. It might be that exercise is not so good, or that you need to modify it significantly, but you won't know until you try it for an extended period of time.

The primary message is for people who think there is no hope in dealing with arthritis. There *is* hope, if you open yourself up to a positive mental attitude. Why let some external source tell you what you can and cannot do when in reality only you can say for sure? You're the one who can push yourself toward the goals you wish to attain. But you have to *want* to be successful. You have to want to put time and effort into your goals and beliefs. It means not settling for second best. It means not having doubts about anything you want to accomplish in your life.

I don't want to limit the message of hope to people with arthritis. Anyone can benefit from a positive mental attitude. Since developing arthritis I've discovered the amazing number of people who have negative attitudes about life in general. They are fearful of trying because they don't want to risk failure. Why? Because they don't have confidence. They aren't in a positive environment that breeds success. You have to surround yourself with encouraging factors in order to deal with your situation in a positive fashion.

I refused to accept second best. I refused to listen to the doctor at Hoag who told me to go home and lie down and get some rest. The last time I did that I was practically paralyzed. If someone is always telling you what you can and cannot do in life, why bother going on? Why don't *you* tell yourself what you can do? And then put your actions where your thoughts are—"Hey, I'm going to go for it." All successful people have one thing in common: they tell themselves, "I'm going to try my best. If I fail, I fail. But if I succeed then that's the highest thing I could have ever done—taking a chance."

When I told Dr. Curd what I wanted to do and he said he'd help me, that's all I needed to hear. I just needed that one little boost and I was on my way. That's what I am hoping this book does. I want it to give people with chronic illness that one boost they might need. I did it, but there is no secret or "magic bullet." It was just plain old hard work. But it happened, and it can work for you.

We all have choices. One of the fundamental choices is choosing to be the best you can be or choosing to be less. That's the first choice you make when you get arthritis. And that's what I'm seeing as *not* being done. There are too many followers and not enough leaders—mentally. People just listen to authority figures and assume they know best. My experience has been that they don't always know what's best. You can turn the control of your life over to the disease, or the doctor, or you can choose to take control of it yourself. The bottom line is that you're never going to know what you are capable of doing unless you try.

What I'm talking about here really goes way beyond arthritis. I've used the Ironman as a metaphor for dealing with this disease. But I'm also using my struggle with arthritis as an analogy for dealing with life in general. This is what it's all about. It's what's up here between our shoulders. How can we best use that to make our lives better?

I don't mean this to sound melodramatic or mystical, but arthritis has presented an opportunity for me to awaken my inner self and to illuminate the big questions in life: Who am I? Where am I going? Why are we here? What does it all mean? Being struck down at a young age, and lying there immobile in bed, really gave me time to think about these big questions. And I came up with some answers. We are not here to be mediocre. We are not here just to survive. We are not here just to go through the motions of life. A tragedy like arthritis can be turned into a positive experience in self-exploration and assertiveness, in creativity and boldness. Each of us has the ability to make a statement, and this book is mine; but its statement is not self-serving—its statement is that we can all make statements.

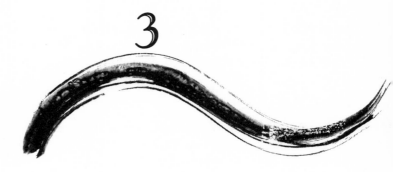

What Is Arthritis and What Can You Do About It?

Arthritis is a very common ailment, yet is vastly misunderstood. It is the subject of an abundant folklore, many half-truths, and a thriving quackery business. Perhaps the most harmful popular belief is the notion that nothing can be done for someone in whom arthritis appears. To the contrary, prompt and continuing treatment can bring many forms of this disease under control."

—FROM *UNDERSTANDING ARTHRITIS* BY THE ARTHRITIS FOUNDATION

The first and most important thing to consider in taking the physical challenge of arthritis is a fundamental, scientifically based, no-nonsense understanding of the disease. Arthritis must be de-mythologized in order to be detected, deduced, and defeated. Dispelling myths is best done through examining data. In other words, as Sergeant Friday said, "Just the facts, Ma'am."

THE BASICS

Consider the facts. More than 37 million Americans (one in seven people and one in three families) have some form of the more than 100 types of arthritis, and the figure is growing by over 200,000 new cases each year. The disease strikes individuals of all ages, from older adults to young children, including over 250,000 under the age of 18. The three most well-known forms of arthritis—osteo, rheumatoid, and gout—account for 16 million, 6.5 million, and 1.6 million arthritis sufferers respectively. Since there is no cure for arthritis, both the absolute and relative numbers of people with the disease continue to grow. Arthritis accounts for more than 27 million lost workdays and 525 million restricted activity days each year. Its cost to the United States economy is approximately $13.8 billion, including $4.4 billion in hospital and nursing home services, $4.8 billion in lost wages, $1.3 billion in lost homemaker services, nearly $1 billion in lost income taxes, and so on, annually.

Because of the lack of proper education about the disease, almost $1 billion are spent annually on questionable "cures" and "remedies." That's 25 dollars for every one dollar in scientific research. People are more interested in immediate cures than in long-term understanding.

In what has traditionally been considered primarily an area of physical disorder, psychological components are now being recognized as important. Couples in which one spouse is arthritic are three times more likely to get divorced. Depression is common at some point in most arthritis sufferers. Anger, anxiety, loss of confidence and self-esteem, and overall feelings of the breakdown of mental health often accompany the disease.

Symptoms

The Arthritis Foundation notes that typical symptoms of arthritis include:

Swelling in one or more joints

Early-morning stiffness

Recurring pain or tenderness in any joint

Inability to move a joint normally

Obvious redness and warmth in a joint

Unexplained weight loss, fever, or weakness combined with joint pain

Symptoms like these persisting for more than two weeks

If you suspect any of these symptoms might be affecting you, consult your doctor immediately. It is very important in developing a program for dealing with arthritis that you come into contact not only with others who suffer as you do, but with *informed* others who can offer sound advice backed by scientific evidence—not people who offer old wives' tales and other forms of nonscientific interpretations of causes and cures. It is vital to be diagnosed and treated as soon as possible so you minimize damage to your joints.

The Nondiscriminatory Disease

The most common misconception about arthritis is that it is an "old people's" disease. That's why no one thought of arthritis when they first wheeled me into the hospital. It is important to remember that arthritis is a nondiscriminatory disease. It has no age barriers—it can happen to young people, individuals in their 20s, or even babies who may be born with it as an almost purely genetic cause. When we think of arthritis we think of our grandmother hunched over when she walks because she is so crippled with arthritis. But our perceptions are wrong. Arthritis can occur anytime, to anyone. It may be more likely to happen to older people, simply because they've been around longer to experience the environmental trigger for their genetic predisposition, but remember that there are nearly 40 million Americans with arthritis and a good portion of them are not what we would call elderly.

Types of Arthritis

Since there are over 100 types of arthritis it would be impossible to cover them all adequately in this chapter, so I will review some of the most common types including osteoarthritis, rheumatoid, lupus, ankylosing spondylitis, gout, scleroderma, and juvenile. I will also briefly examine infectious arthritis, bursitis, and tendinitis.

OSTEOARTHRITIS.   The most common form of arthritis, osteoarthritis does not attack the entire body, but is specific to certain joints and is caused by a wearing down of the protective cartilage until eventually the bone itself is attacked. The most common joints affected are fingers, hips, knees, and the spine. Osteoarthritis is more related to age than many other forms of arthritis, and thus may be the result of time- and stress-related causes such as excessive wear in athletes, physical workers, and so on. Osteoarthritis is predominantly found in women. As the thin sheath that normally protects the joints (by acting as a lubricant) gets worn away or deteriorates, you end up with bone against bone. It's like taking two pieces of sandpaper and grinding them together.

RHEUMATOID ARTHRITIS.   Rheumatoid arthritis typically strikes between the ages of 20 and 55 and focuses on the joints of the hands, feet, arms, legs, and hips. The latest evidence points to genetic markers that predispose an individual to be more susceptible to this, an autoimmune disease. It is believed that the cause is a derangement of the body's self-defense or autoimmune system in which inflammation of the joints is caused by the body essentially attacking itself. What is attacked initially is the synovial membranes of the joints, which are normally lubricating for smooth action of joint movement. The inflammation can then spread into the cartilage of the joints, causing deformation, restriction of motion, and extreme pain. If the hands are affected, the fingers can become distorted. In rheumatoid arthritis it's not the bones that hurt, but the area around the bones. It becomes so inflamed that it stiffens you up. The inflamed muscles then press on the nerves and tendons, and that pressure is what hurts. In that limited joint space you are increasing the amount of mass inside, which increases the pressure. It's like crimping a straw and trying to blow through it.

LUPUS.   Most of the 400,000 Americans with systemic lupus erythematosus are women in their child-bearing years. Lupus is characterized by damage to the skin, joints, and internal organs. Symptoms include fever, muscle aches, skin rash, swollen glands, loss of weight, weakness, nausea, fatigue, joint pain, and anemia. It is not unusual for nerve and brain damage to also occur. Like rheumatoid arthritis, lupus may be triggered by a genetic marker that turns the immune system against the body.

ANKYLOSING SPONDYLITIS.   This spinal disease attacks the joints of the spine, causing inflammation and, in extreme cases, fusing them together. Men between the ages of 20 and 40 are commonly affected, and show such symptoms as low back pain and stiffness that continue for months. Generally, especially in milder cases, the symptoms will subside, especially if treated early with anti-inflammatory drugs and special exercises.

GOUT.   Known in the 19th century as the "rich-man's disease" because of its association with "rich" foods, gout is now known to be caused by an increase in uric acid in the synovial fluid that surrounds cartilage. It can be controlled by medication. Gout can attack any joint of the body, but in 75 percent of the cases it is the big toe that is attacked. The excess uric acids causes needle-like crystals to form in the joints, which, in turn, cause inflammation. It is the only form of arthritis that is consistently affected by diet.

SCLERODERMA.   Scleroderma, translated as "hard skin," is a systemic disease that, like rheumatoid arthritis, can affect the entire body. Inflammation of internal organs can occur in addition to the hardening and thickening of the skin. Women more than men are affected, and the age ranges for susceptibility are between 40 and 50. There is no known cause and most suffer from only mild symptoms.

JUVENILE.   Affecting a quarter of a million children nationwide, juvenile arthritis may include rheumatoid, lupus, ankylosing spondylitis, and others, with various symptoms that include rash, fever, inflammation of the eyes, fatigue, and swelling of the muscles and joints. Because they are still growing, children with symptoms should be diagnosed immediately and treated before permanent joint damage occurs. Many forms of juvenile arthritis go into remission within months or years, though some continue into adulthood.

INFECTIOUS ARTHRITIS.   Not to be mistaken as a contagious form of arthritis, rather infectious arthritis is caused by complications from viral, bacterial, or fungal infections. The infectious agent triggers the initial disease, which then attacks the joints, inducing the onset of arthritis. Gonorrhea, for example, can also cause arthritis. Elimination of the original infection often terminates the arthritis.

BURSITIS AND TENDINITIS. Temporary forms of arthritis caused by excessive stress on a joint, bursitis is the inflammation of a bursa, or small sac between a tendon and bone, while tendinitis is the inflammation of a tendon. Rest or a change of activities will often eliminate inflammation and pain.

Causes of Arthritis

As you can see, the list of types of arthritis is long and varied, and we've only scratched the surface. To think that there is *a* cause of arthritis is as misleading as thinking there is *a* cause of cancer. The causes of arthritis are varied, complicated, and not fully understood, despite the claims of many books on the market. There are many theories coming into vogue, but it is important to remember that no one just "has" arthritis. You have to ask what *type* of arthritis before you can even discuss the cause. In my case, I have both ankylosing spondylitis and Reiter's syndrome, possibly caused by a genetic predisposition for arthritis that was later triggered environmentally by rheumatic fever when I was 21 years old. When I had rheumatic fever I was hospitalized with a temperature of 104 degrees. I was ready to "check out." My doctors think that this is what might have been the environmental stimulus for my arthritis. I've even been genetically checked by doctors and I have a genetic marker for rheumatoid arthritis, meaning I am genetically predisposed to develop the disease. No one in my immediate family has arthritis, but it can skip generations.

So on a very general level, most forms of arthritis are caused by both genetics and environment, even though in my case it was years and years after that disease that the arthritis attacked my body. Since there are so many types of arthritis, there can be a wide variety of environmental triggers—different for different people. As we saw, for example, gout can be triggered by certain foods, given that the individual is already disposed to get gout.

Therefore, it is vital that you get properly informed by the best medical and scientific people in the field, before you try to draw any conclusions about your disease.

ARTHRITIS AND TREATMENT

The fact of the matter is, scientifically speaking, there is no cure for most of the forms of arthritis, though modern medical research has made and continues to make some progress. Genetic markers have been discovered that indicate the potential for certain types of arthritis. As noted above, the immune system seems to be the culprit in rheumatoid arthritis, and work is being done in bolstering the body's natural defenses and preventing it from attacking the body it is supposed to defend.

Treatment, not Cures

Instead of discussing cures, medical doctors and health practitioners approach the disease with treatments. Most treatment therapies traditionally deal with drugs—pain-killers and anti-inflammatory drugs. That has always been the main form of treatment, along with "lots of rest." But in the last five or six years exercise therapy and an active lifestyle have become a recognized part of dealing with the disease. Before, exercise was generally prohibited, or at least not recommended, because most medical doctors felt that exercise would inflame the area and increase the amount of pain. But now we're finding out that exercise is a very positive part of therapy, both physically and mentally. Exercise keeps the joints loose and mobile.

In general, the basic goals of the various forms of treatment are the attenuation of pain and the accentuation of mobility. These include:

Rest and relaxation
Exercise
Use of heat and cold
Joint protection
Self-help aids
Medications
Surgery

Most suggestions for dealing with arthritis involve protecting your joints, avoiding painful situations, and increasing your efficiency in moving about the environment. For example, here are a number of suggestions for making your life easier:

LISTEN TO YOUR BODY. Pain, for example, is often a warning mechanism. If it hurts too much, then back off. (Sometimes pain is an indication of something good you are doing in the form of strength building—more on this later.)

BE AWARE OF STRESSFUL BODY POSITIONS. Some positions are better than others for relieving stress. Leaning on one arm or leg or tightly gripping something with your fingers can cause extra stress on the joints.

CONTROL YOUR WEIGHT. More weight means more stress on your joints, particularly in your lower back, hips, and knees.

DON'T STAY IN ONE POSITION CONTINUOUSLY. If you keep moving, you keep your joints moving and the fluid in the joints does not build up.

TAKE ADVANTAGE OF YOUR STRONGEST JOINTS AND MUSCLES. Women could carry a purse over their shoulder rather than hold it in their hand. Push open doors or close drawers with your shoulder or hip instead of your fingers. When using stairs lead with your stronger leg going up and your weaker leg going down. When you lift heavy objects, bend your knees and pick them up with your legs, not your back.

SIMPLIFY YOUR WORK AND HOME.   The Arthritis Foundation has publications that list hundreds of things you can do around the home and office to make it easier to get around and protect your joints.

Medications

Though none will cure, there are some medications that will help decrease inflammation or the pain or arthritis.

ASPIRIN.   The wonder drug of the 20th century, aspirin also helps arthritis in a number of ways, including pain relief and inflammation control. It is cheap, readily available from almost any store, and has relatively few side effects, with the exception of repeated large dosages causing stomach irritation in some people.

GOLD TREATMENTS.   No one knows exactly how it works, but for some people—and it differs from individual to individual—gold treatments in the form of pills or injections seem to reduce the pain of rheumatoid arthritis.

IMMUNOSUPPRESSIVE DRUGS.   In the case where the immune system appears to be the cause of the destruction of the joint, these drugs weaken the body cells that produce the immune and inflammatory action. Because of serious side effects (including the possibility of cancer) these drugs are recommended only when nearly all else has been tried.

CORTICOSTEROIDS. These cortisone-related drugs are good for reducing inflammation during acute flare-ups, though they also are known to cause serious side effects.

PENICILLAMINE. Related to penicillin (though with different effects), this drug is only used under a physician's supervision, and only when other methods have been tried. Results thus far are tentative and months of experimenting are needed to see any effect.

IL-IRA. Medical research continues to explore new possibilities that could help arthritis sufferers. For example, a Boulder, Colorado-based biotechnology company, *Synergen*, has recently announced in the *Wall Street Journal* that they have found a protein that the body uses to turn off the inflammation-producing mechanism that causes the pain of arthritis. The protein, called *IL-ira*, in laboratory tests on animals "blocked inflammation and even stopped some bone destruction caused by severe arthritis." *IL-ira* is thought to be the chemical that turns off another immune-system substance called interleukin-1, or *IL-1*. People with arthritis have more than the normal amount of *IL-1*. It is thought that *IL-1* triggers the production of a chemical that fights infection from bacteria. An excessive amount of this chemical in joints causes swelling, inflammation, and pain. Further research remains to be done on *IL-ira* and its possible side effects, which could include the reduction of immunity to other forms of bacteria.

Medical and Other Specialists

One of the first questions you will have to answer, if you are uncertain about having arthritis, or what to do about it if you do, is "what kind of doctor should I see?" The answer, of course, depends on what knowledge you have of your condition. If you have symptoms but are uncertain whether or not it is arthritis, then you should begin with your family doctor, who is likely a general practitioner. He or she can at least make an initial diagnosis, and then recommend a specialist. Specialists abound, and if you've had arthritis for awhile, you've probably already been through the gamut of choices. They include:

ORTHOPEDISTS: Doctors who specialize in diseases of the bones and joints would be the kind to see if you obtain the diagnosis of osteoarthritis. Orthopedists would perform surgery, if deemed necessary.

OSTEOPATHS: Doctors of osteopathy, or diseases of the bones, may use manipulation of bones and joints in addition to traditional medicine.

RHEUMATOLOGISTS: Medical doctors who specialize in rheumatic conditions, rheumatologists diagnose and treat rheumatoid and other types of arthritis.

NEUROLOGISTS AND NEUROSURGEONS: Specialists in the nervous system and its disorders, neurologists and neurosurgeons deal with related diseases and injuries that affect pain in the patient.

PHYSIATRISTS AND PHYSICAL THERAPISTS: Specialists in physical therapy and rehabilitation, physiatrists and physical therapists work with patients on strength, flexibility, range of motion, and pain control.

EXERCISE AND HEALTH THERAPISTS: These therapists develop an exercise or training program individually tailored for the patient's program of rehabilitation. They will recommend gyms, exercise machines, and specific daily, weekly, monthly, and yearly programs for recovery.

CHIROPRACTORS: Chiropractors are trained in spinal and joint manipulation for pain relief, with emphasis on the relationship of structure and functions of the body.

ACUPUNCTURISTS: Acupuncturists are practitioners in pain control and relief through acupuncture, the insertion of needles at specific points in the body. Although much controversy surrounds the validity of both its theory and practice, many arthritic patients report both short-term and long-term relief from pain.

ACUPRESSURISTS AND MASSAGE THERAPISTS: These rehabilitation and recovery specialists are trained in manipulation of muscles, tendons, and joints through massage and pressure (as opposed to the chiropractic methods of more sudden manipulation of the spine and joints).

PSYCHOLOGISTS AND PSYCHIATRISTS: These specialists in mental processes may assist in pain control, emotional difficulties in dealing with the disease, family complications surrounding the disease, and general support in meeting the mental challenge of arthritis.

OCCUPATIONAL THERAPISTS: Occupational therapists assist you in getting back on your feet, both at home and in the work place, by offering advice on ways to deal with pain and inflammation and still function in the work force and at home.

When you first encounter doctors as an arthritis patient, they are at the very least extremely cautious and even a bit on the pessimistic side. Because arthritis is so varied, it really comes down to each and every individual person as to how he or she should be treated. For example, I went to see my doctor about a week and a half ago, and I hadn't seen him in almost four years. He told me, "George, there are people who have the exact same disease you have, yet they have made practically no progress at all."

Why? Because arthritis is as much a part of the mind as it is the body. It is the mental game. It's your attitude. My doctor told me, "I always think about you when I see people who have a down attitude and say, 'Oh, I can't do anything because I hurt too much' and all that—they are limiting themselves." The reason for this is that they don't let the old, negative mental processes go and let in the new, positive mental processes. But this is just what you must do—and believe me, the results are worth it.

THE MENTAL GAME

Since I've had this disease I've become much more aware of how negative people can be about themselves and life. There are very few optimists in this world. There are a lot of pessimists who never reach their best, or make their highest goals, because they always doubt what they are doing, or doubt the world, or doubt their environment. They never realize that there is a wealth of opportunity out there to be what you want to be—to accomplish any goal you want to accomplish, if you just believe in yourself and have the right attitude. Also, since I've had this disease, I've recognized that people are afraid of success at the same time. They are afraid of trying because they think, "If I try I might fail." So fear of success is really fear of failure—they go hand in hand. Because they are fearful of not succeeding they are guaranteeing failure. They've preconditioned themselves to this fear-of-failure mode in their thinking and they never get out of it. But there is hope. There is the possibility of living a full and active life.

Mental versus Physical

The medical community does not really address the mental issue in arthritis, or most diseases for that matter. Yet I don't point a finger at anyone, because after all, the medical community is medical. It deals with drugs and the physical body. The problem with this unilinear approach is that people are then programmed that the pill will be the quick fix to their problem—the magic elixir. Although the medical community realizes the importance of the mental game, our society is so caught up in the "quick-fix" syndrome that it applies pressure to doctors to treat patients medically, or physically, ignoring the psychological aspects. The mental challenge of arthritis is *working* at this problem. It's not taking a pill and magically becoming better. Don't think you are going to go out tomorrow and do something, either physically or mentally, and you will be better. Arthritis is not that type of disease.

You have to draw up a game plan of how you work with your disease. You have to plan for a long game. It's a stepping-stone procedure that's both physical and mental. It's a balance between the mind and the body. That's what this book is about—balancing the physical challenge with the mental challenge. Most readers will be looking for books on how to deal with arthritis physically—I know because I was one of them—but what I discovered was that it is the mental challenge that counts at least as much, if not more.

My uncle is a perfect example. He has gout. He is 55 years old and he is overweight, drinks a lot of beer, never exercises, and doesn't feel good. He looks at me and says "You sure look good," as if it were some sort of miracle that he has yet to find. He asks me what I do to feel good, and I tell him I exercise every day and keep myself motivated. He sits there with his chin in his gut, not even listening to what I'm saying, because he is used to being told that he can't exercise, that "that's it, just go home and take these pills and maybe you'll feel better and maybe you won't."

This is precisely what attracts people to the "cures" for arthritis. It's drawing for straws, like the lottery. People are attracted to the lottery because they are hoping for that one big strike so they won't have to work anymore. It's like that with arthritis. People are hoping they can just buy a magic potion and they will be cured. But these people are just playing mental hooky. They aren't working at success. They are waiting for the lottery to come their way. But there is no arthritis lottery for anyone to win. People are looking for the easy way out, but there is nothing in life that is worth having that is easy to get, and the same is true of arthritis. You have to work, and that is what makes it all worthwhile—achieving your goals through good, hard work and organization.

DOUBTFUL CLAIMS

Arthritics are one of the prime targets for these miracle-cure proponents. In fact, the Arthritis Foundation estimates that $950 million a year go for questionable remedies.

The reason for the gullibility is that when you're in so much pain you'll do anything for relief. You'll try a lot of stuff to feel better, yet the pain does not subside. It just keeps going and going and going and there is no relief. You'll try anything people tell you. "Well, try this special herb tea. It will help." You try it and it doesn't work. That's just quackery. But what sometimes happens is that someone will try one of these touted remedies and "get better." The real explanation is that the disease goes in and out and by chance, that someone tried the latest miracle cure during one of these remission phases, attributing his success to that potion.

Believe me, I've been through all the magic elixir books where you drink the "raspberry root tea" with the "buckthorn bark root" and that is supposed to make you better. I've tried the 14 enemas a day, colonics, the whole deal. I've tried virtually everything there is to try, and none of them works. Save yourself a lot of time and money and take my word for it—there is no magic cure. You'll be tempted because the pain is so bad, but one of the advantages of educating yourself on the disease is that you'll find many others who have already tried all these things and they'll all tell you the same thing—they don't work. The Arthritis Foundation has compiled the following list of things that are unknown, harmless, or even harmful:

Unknown:
Bee venom
Biofeedback
Diets
Fish oil
Lasers
Vaccine therapy
Yucca

Harmless:
Acupuncture
Copper bracelets
Mineral springs
Spas
Topical creams
Uranium
Vibrators
Vinegar and honey

Harmful:
DMSO (A horse liniment used by athletes in the 1970s for injuries.)
Large doses of vitamins
Snake venom
Drugs with hidden ingredients

A good general rule of thumb in watching out for doubtful panaceas is that they are probably promising the thing you want most—to completely rid yourself of arthritis. The following are clues that the remedy should probably be avoided:

Claims to work for all types of arthritis as well as other health problems. Since arthritis consists of over 100 types, this is impossible.

Evidence is in the form of case histories or testimonials: "I know someone who tried this and they got better." Science depends on controlled experiments, not hearsay.

Cites one study as proof. Science depends on verification from many studies.

Cites a study without a control group. Scientists must compare a treated group with a nontreated group. If Drug X worked for this group of people, then there must be another group of people who didn't take the drug and didn't get better.

Contents are not listed in drug or "remedy."

Is not approved by the FDA or has no information or warnings about side effects.

Is described as a "natural" healer.

Claims it is based on a secret formula. Science depends on validation from other scientists and laboratories. There are no secrets in science.

Is available only from one source: "Available only through this exclusive offer."

Claims it cures arthritis. There are no "cures" for arthritis. When there are, believe me—you will hear about it everywhere!

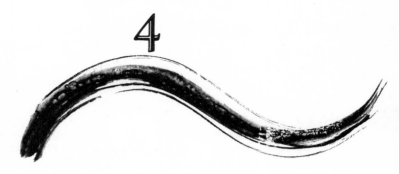

Arthritis and Exercise

"Everyone should be his own physician. We ought to assist, and not force nature."

—Voltaire

      Learning to live with arthritis is the focus of this book, and to this extent exercise is a critically important subject. It certainly embodies the spirit of the physical challenge, and as we shall see, the mental challenge as well.

      For this chapter, getting involved means getting physically active—taking action about your problem. When I made the remark in *Reader's Digest* about taking the problem by the "scruff of the neck," I meant taking action. Here we shall examine the role of exercise in taking action in your arthritis rehabilitation.

TIME TO GET INVOLVED

When I was going through rehabilitation I had a saying that I repeated over and over in my mind. I still remind myself of it today: *T.T.G.I.*, or *Time To Get Involved*. Learning to be a participant again means learning to get involved, both physically and mentally.

Traditional medical advice in years past recommended sufferers of arthritis do nothing physical. This is all changing. My program offers a totally involved, active lifestyle, centered around exercise. Even if it is the minimal amount, relative to your particular strengths and weaknesses, exercise is extremely beneficial for learning to live with arthritis. I want to demonstrate first how exercise is important for both the quality and quantity of life for anyone, including arthritics; and second, why the arthritis sufferer in particular should exercise, and the specific benefits to you in getting into an exercise program.

THE EXERCISE–HEALTH CONNECTION

In 300 B.C. the Greek philosopher Herophilus said: "When health is absent, wisdom cannot become manifest, strength cannot be exerted, wealth is useless and reason is powerless." It's great to be an intellectual, but an intellectual who is also strong physically is a more well-balanced person. So not only did working out physically every day help my arthritis, it also helped my mental state. It gave me confidence because I was physically able to move more easily.

Is there a real connection between exercise and health? There is. For example, in a 1986 article in the *New England Journal of Medicine* the results of a long-term study of 16,936 Harvard University graduates were presented showing conclusively that exercise not only increases health but helps you live longer. In one of the most thorough and comprehensive studies of its kind ever done, the researchers discovered that if you exercise regularly you can expect to live, on the average, two years longer than the sedentary individual.

Specifically, the researchers concluded that those who expend at least 2,000 calories per week exercising (approximately one hour a day of any aerobic exercise including cycling, swimming, jogging, or brisk walking) are more likely to reach the age of 80 than someone who exercises less than 2,000 calories a week. The paper also reported that between ages 40 and 70, for every hour you exercise you will gain two hours of life. By exercising six hours a week (one hour a day with a day off) for 30 years, a 40-year-old will live an extra 18,720 hours, or 780 days—2.14 extra years of life. The paper also had this to say about the connection between exercise and health:

> The reported gains in longevity are averages and could be as high as an extra 20 years for some.
>
> Exercise not only alleviates rheumatoid arthritis symptoms, it also decreases the risk of heart disease, cancer, and osteoporosis.
>
> In this study the benefits of exercise leveled off at 3,500 calories per week, or about 1.5 hours of exercise a day, so you needn't be an exercise fanatic in order to stay healthy.
>
> Research data from Holland was reported, concluding that exercising consistently in small amounts throughout the year was better than seasonal exercising in large amounts. "The strenuousness of the exercise didn't have as much to do with the benefits as being active year-round," the researchers concluded, so you don't even have to exercise all that hard. Consistency is the key.

In addition, exercise has many general health benefits, which include:

Strengthens your heart
Lowers your resting pulse rate

Lowers your blood pressure

Lowers your serum cholesterol levels

Cleanses your pores

Develops your lung capacity

Improves the efficiency of oxygen consumption

Stimulates the production of endorphins, chemical substances in the brain that may reduce the perception of pain

THE EXERCISE—ARTHRITIS CONNECTION

These studies were done without looking specifically at the benefits of exercise on arthritis. Why should someone with arthritis exercise, particularly when it can be painful, and thus seemingly harmful? You should exercise because it has been proven, both scientifically and through anecdotal evidence from thousands of arthritis sufferers, that exercise helps attenuate arthritis symptoms. How? Through the following ways:

Exercise increases the circulation of the blood, which helps keep the joints warm and well-lubricated and thus easier to move.

Exercise increases the range of motion of the legs, arms, fingers, and neck, by stretching the tendons and ligaments.

Exercise increases muscular strength, which for those muscles surrounding joints means greater joint protection.

Exercise increases the production of endorphins, which act as a natural pain control that for arthritics can be especially beneficial.

Exercise strengthens the muscles in the back, which can help straighten your posture.

Exercise prevents you from being too inactive, which may cause the joints to become stiffer and even lock up.

Exercise increases bone strength.

Exercise decreases the chances of getting osteoporosis.

Exercise increases your overall health and well-being, making you feel more positive about yourself. If you look good, you feel good. Physical action breeds mental action. It gets you moving, both physically and mentally.

It is important to note here that exercise may not always be good. In fact, being an arthritis sufferer has taught me to measure my exercise with a solid dose of rest each day. And, of course, there are days when I don't exercise at all, though these are very rare. This will vary from person to person.

Time to Rest

The importance of rest lies in a balance between exercise and non-exercise depending on the current condition of your arthritis. During flare-ups of arthritic pain and inflammation doctors usually recommend more rest and less exercise; and vice versa when the symptoms seem to be in remission. While I would agree with this on one level, on another you have to do what is right for you. There is no "meter" to measure how bad your arthritis is at the doctor's office. Pain and your perception of it are what count. I would suggest experimenting with exercise at *all* times, and then taper off if it turns out to be hurting, rather than helping, your long-range performance. During these flare-ups you might even experiment with having shorter periods of exercise several times during the day rather than one long one. This might help maintain mobility all day long. More on balance will be discussed in chapter 10.

Your Daily Checklist

When I was in the hospital I kept thinking to myself, what can I do to get out of this bed? What can I do to move again? When you are an arthritic, you have to keep moving. Some days when you wake up you are stiff and sore and a little locked up. You have to go through your daily checklist before you begin exercising. When you get up each day mentally go through your physical checklist:

How are my joints?
How are my muscles?
How are my knees?
How is my back?
How are my shoulders?
How are my arms?
How is my neck?

And so on. It's like each day is starting over again when you get up. The bed is the place to rest. When you are through resting, it's time to start moving again but you've got to make sure that each joint is ready. It pays to take just a little extra time each morning getting started, especially if this is when you are doing your exercise program.

BEGINNING AN EXERCISE PROGRAM

The first thing you should do is consult your doctor, and go through a rehabilitation center that knows and understands the arthritic condition. Sports-medicine doctors also tend to be quite knowledgeable about joint movement and joint problems, including arthritis. The appendix at the end of the book has a list of the Arthritis Foundation Chapters around the United States. Before beginning an exercise program, contact your local chapter and get the names of some doctors, physical therapists, or sports-medicine trainers that have knowledge and experience in working with arthritis patients.

Establishing a Base Level

Next, you've got to establish what your physical abilities are. In order to design a complete exercise program, you must know at what level to begin. The last thing you want to do is just walk into a gym and grab the first set of barbells and start "pumping iron." You will likely pump yourself right back to the doctor. A good trainer will have you check the following two important characteristics:

RANGE OF MOTION.   This refers to the extent to which a joint can be moved through its normal range. For example, how far can you push your head toward your left shoulder or your right shoulder? Can you touch your chin to your chest? How far back can you tilt your head? These are questions regarding the range of motion of your neck. You should also check the range of motion of your feet, your legs, your arms, your hands, and your fingers. A therapist will make a note of the *degree* of the range of motion, with which you can make later comparisons.

If you don't have someone to do this for you, you can make a note for each area and go through the motion exercises yourself. For example, for your arms you might stand sideways next to a wall and lift your arm straight up, noting with a pencil how far up you were able to raise it. Check this each day or week as you progress in your exercises, to see how your range of motion is doing. You can do the same thing with your legs by lying on the floor, sideways against the wall, then seeing how high you can lift your leg. Mark that point with a pencil so you can check it periodically. Stretching exercises will help increase your range of motion.

STRENGTH OF MUSCLE GROUPS.   Check the strength of each of your limbs, specific muscle groups, and even specific muscles. You should literally make charts to keep track of what level you were when you began, and how those levels change over time. Not all gyms have the same equipment, so you will need to establish one place to work out, get tested on those machines and be consistent in working on those machines as you slowly increase your levels of strength. Since everyone suffers setbacks, any decreases in muscle strength can be analyzed so you can determine if you are doing something differently in your workout, nutrition, or lifestyle in general that may be having an adverse effect. Then you can change it in order to get back to your previous higher level.

Virtually all gyms will supply you with a chart that lists each machine, with places to write in your initial weight levels. There should be blank spaces for you to write in the new numbers as you get stronger.

STRETCHING

After you've established where you are physically, your therapist will help you design a program at each level to reach the next highest one. The first level is usually stretching and range of motion exercises. Warming-up—stretching—is one of the most important things any arthritic can do. Permanent joint deformity may result from a lack of proper range of motion exercises. Sometimes a joint can even get stuck in a bent position, called a flexion contracture. Stretching will prevent such contractures.

Anyone can learn to stretch, regardless of age or amount of flexibility. Often we watch the incredibly limber gymnasts contorting themselves into human knots, and we groan in sympathetic pain. In stretching, though, all things are relative. If, in touching your toes, you feel the same amount of tautness and pain in your muscles at mid-calf as someone else does when touching the ground, those are equal stretches, relative to the body doing the stretch. For arthritics, for whom stiffness can be a daily problem, starting the day off with stretching can be critical to a comfortable, pain-free day.

Why Should You Stretch?

To relax the muscles

To keep muscles loose and supple

To stretch tendons and ligaments

To increase range of motion in all joints

To improve circulation

To help prevent muscle injuries such as tears and strains

To help prevent joint injuries by exceeding the range of motion

To heighten psychological awareness of the body's working parts

When Should You Stretch?

In the morning, before the start of the day's activities

During breaks at work to relieve muscle tension in the neck and back

After sitting or standing for long periods of time

Before any physically taxing activity—not necessarily just sports—for instance, working around the yard, walking, hiking, or moving furniture

During an athletic event, if there is a lull in the action, to keep the muscles supple and loose

Anytime you feel like it while doing activities such as watching television or listening to music

How Should You Stretch?

Stretching should be done slowly, without bouncing or jerky movements. Stretch to the point where you feel a slight tension in the muscle, then slowly increase the stretch until you feel a slight pain. Do not stretch until it hurts beyond reason. The slight pain is just an indication that the muscle is taut. Hold this slight stretch for 15–30 seconds, then slowly release it. Try it again and this time attempt to stretch a little beyond the previous point.

Proper breathing is very important in stretching. Your breathing should be slow, rhythmical, and under control. Exhale while you are going into a stretch; inhale while coming out of a stretch. Do not hold your breath during the stretch. Breathe consistently during the 15- to 30-second stretch.

Stretching is not an athletic contest. It isn't considered "macho" by any athletes to be able to stretch into various contorted positions. The key to successful stretching is to be relaxed. Don't worry about flexibility; if you stretch relaxed, flexibility will come. It's just one of the many positive results of regular stretching.

It may seem at first to be a time-consuming nuisance to have to go through the routine every day or each time you exercise. But once you get into the habit, stretching really becomes a part of your daily life, and it feels wrong to begin without it.

STRENGTH TRAINING

The next thing to work on is strength. Doing specific exercises to strengthen specific groups of muscles can be established at any decent gym, and there are even plenty of exercises you can do at home in case you don't want to join a gym or are not near one. The important thing is to not go about this in some haphazard manner. That's how injuries occur, and injuries to an arthritic are magnified considerably because of the brittleness of the joints and bones. Each training program must be custom designed to fit the individual. Each arthritic patient is different, with different strengths and weaknesses.

Find a gym that is equipped with modern weight machines, has a pleasant atmosphere with clean and spacious workout areas and locker rooms, and is fully staffed with knowledgeable instructors. It is best to find a gym close to your home or workplace so you are less likely to skip a session. Go to gyms that offer trial visits and ask members what they think. Weigh their recommendations against your observations before making a final decision.

How to Begin Strength Training

When you are ready to begin, set aside consistent time blocks of 45–90 minutes per day, three days per week. Set goals for yourself and do the exercises, allowing at least one day between workouts for recovery. Remember to take it easy at the start, beginning with the weights that were established for your base levels. Exercising too vigorously will cause soreness and quickly sour your attitude toward strength training. Stay in tune with your body. In addition, learn to breathe properly. The basic rule is to exhale when reaching the point of greatest resistance and inhale when hitting the place of least resistance. Gradually this breathing pattern will come naturally.

Wear comfortable clothing that allows you to move without restriction. Outfits made from cotton or other natural fibers absorb perspiration, dry quickly, and are easy to care for.

Monitor your workouts by keeping a training log. Write down the repetitions, the number of sets, the number of pounds you lift, and try to describe what is happening to your body. Refer to your training log frequently; it will provide encouragement when you become discouraged about your progress.

The Well-planned Workout

At each station at the gym it is best to do two or three sets of each exercise. Complete the full routine, one set at each station, then repeat. Some people prefer to do all their sets at a station before moving on. Either way is acceptable, though the former may provide a little more variety and thus prevent overworking one set of muscles and joints at one time.

After starting at the base levels of weight, slowly and systematically increase them as the weeks and months go by. If you suffer persistent pain and stress in your joints, decrease the amount or type of exercise rather than try to be "macho" by forcing the motion.

Strength training exercises are depicted in the following photos, each with a brief descriptive caption. These are some of the exercises I did during my rehabilitation, and that I still do to maintain my strength and flexibility.

ENDURANCE TRAINING

Once you have mobility and strength, you need to work on endurance. By endurance I mean the ability to be able to sustain a reasonably active lifestyle throughout the day without getting really tired or run-down. You may have good strength, but if your endurance is low then you will get more tired at the end of the day and be more susceptible to injuries. Swimming, jogging, cycling, or any activity that increases your cardiovascular fitness is beneficial to endurance. How? Increasing your heart and breathing rate makes the cardiovascular system stronger, and thus more efficient.

How much do you need to increase it? You need to increase your heart rate to within your "target heart zone" approximately 30 to 60 minutes a day. Your "target heart zone" is easily calculated by subtracting your age from 220, then multiplying by .60 and .75. The results are your "target heart zone" numbers. For example, if you are 50 years of age, the calculation would be as follows:

$$
\begin{array}{r}
220 \\
-\ 50 \\
\hline
170
\end{array}
\qquad
\begin{array}{r}
170 \\
\times\ .60 \\
\hline
102
\end{array}
\qquad
\begin{array}{r}
170 \\
\times\ .75 \\
\hline
128
\end{array}
$$

So 102 to 128 is the target heart zone for a 50-year-old person. Your pulse rate can be calculated by counting the number of beats in your neck's carotid artery for 6 seconds, then multiplying this number by 10. To be more accurate, count for 10 seconds, then multiply the number by 6. See the chart below for easy reference. To find the carotid artery place two fingers at the back of your jaw and slide them down onto your neck. You should feel your pulse beating fairly strongly.

TARGET HEART RATE CHART

Age	Target Heart Rate	10-second count
20	120–150	20–25
25	117–146	19–24
30	114–143	19–24
35	111–139	18–23
40	108–135	18–23
45	105–131	17–22
50	102–128	17–21
55	99–124	16–21
60	96–120	16–20
65	93–116	15–19
70	90–113	15–19
75	87–109	14–18
80	84–105	14–18
85	81–101	13–17

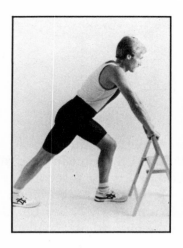 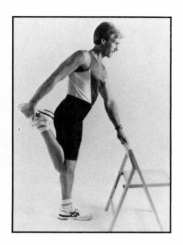

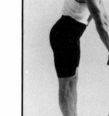

Photography:
Bryson Martin

The weight
system courtesy
of Spenco Fitness

Figure 1. *Calf Stretch.* Leaning against a chair, keep your heel flat to the ground and lean forward, stretching your right calf. Hold the stretch for 20 seconds, then switch legs.

Figure 2. *Thigh Stretch.* Steady yourself against the chair while you pull your right leg up toward your rear, feeling the stretch in your thigh. Hold this stretch for 20 seconds, then switch legs.

Figure 3. *Shin Stretch.* Steady yourself against the chair, then rock back on your heels, keeping your knees straight and locked so that you feel the stretch in your shins. Hold for 15 seconds.

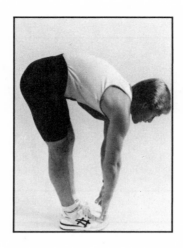

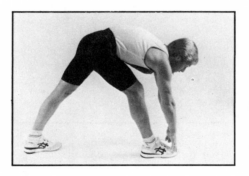

Figure 4a and 4b. *Toe Touch.* Keeping your feet flat on the ground, reach down with your arms straight and your fingers out and touch your toes. Hold for 30 seconds. If you can't touch your toes, keep your feet flat and knees straight and reach as far as possible. If this is particularly difficult, you can try touching your toes with one leg forward and the other back, as demonstrated in the second photo. In time you will be able to touch your toes.

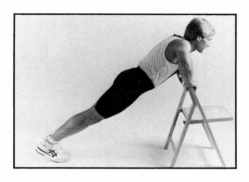

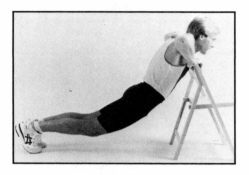

Figure 5. *Double Calf Stretch.* Same procedure as the *Calf Stretch,* but hold for 30 seconds.

Figure 6. *Back and Shoulder Stretch.* Holding yourself against the chair, curl your body down toward the floor without touching the floor with your knees. Hold for 15 seconds. This will not only stretch and loosen your lower back, it will flex and loosen your shoulders and arms.

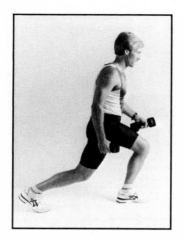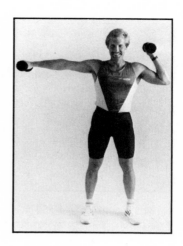

Figure 7. *Thigh Flex.* Holding the weights at your side, lean forward keeping your left leg ahead and your right leg behind, then alternate legs every 5 seconds, back and forth 20 times.

Figure 8. *Bicep Stretch.* Begin by holding the weights straight out, then curl one up toward your shoulder, then back straight out while you curl the other one up toward your shoulder, and so on back and forth. Begin with 10 repetitions and then work up.

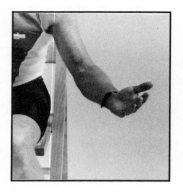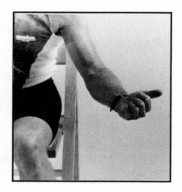

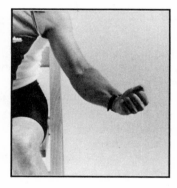

Figure 9a, 9b, and 9c. *Finger Curls.* Sitting in a relaxed position, stretch your fingers straight out, then curl them up into a fist, as pictured, then stretch the fingers back out, and so on, slowly, 20 times. Switch hands and do 20 repetitions. If you can, repeat three times for each hand.

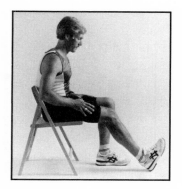
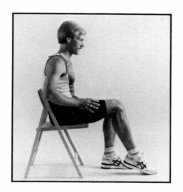
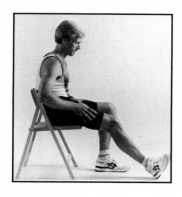

Figure 10a, 10b, and 10c. *Foot and Ankle Stretch.* Sitting on the chair, stretch one leg forward, heel on the ground with your toes pointing up, move your foot left and right, and then around in circles, keeping your heel on the ground. Switch legs and repeat. Then do the same exercise with your toes on the ground, heel up, and rock the heel left and right, and then around in circles, keeping your toes on the ground. Do for 30 seconds in each position.

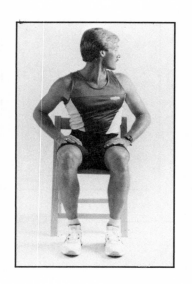 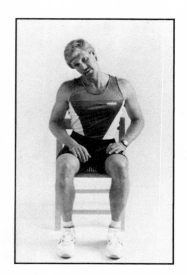

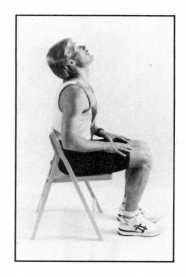

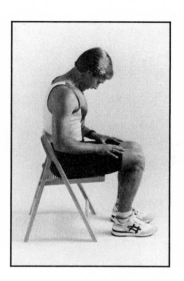

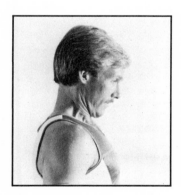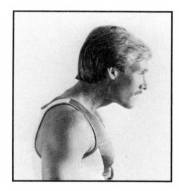

Figure 11a, 11b, 11c, 11d, 11e, and 11f. *Neck Stretch.* Sitting on the chair with your hand on your thighs, stretch your neck slowly left, then right, 20 times; then rock your head toward your shoulders, left, then right, 20 times; then stretch your head backwards, then forwards, 20 times; then, keeping your shoulders and head straight, touch your chin to your chest, then stretch your chin straight out, then back to your chest, and so on 20 times.

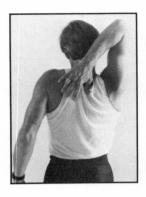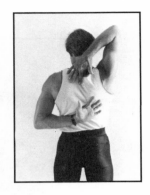

Figure 12a and 12b. *Shoulder Stretch*. With your feet flat on the ground and your left arm straight at your side, reach behind your head and touch between your shoulder blade, stretching as far as possible. If you can't touch your back, just go as far as possible, and hold for 15 seconds. Switch arms. Repeat with other arm placed behind back.

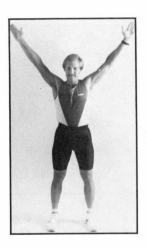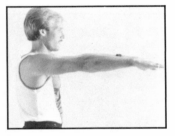

Figure 13a and 13b. *Arm and Shoulder Stretch*. Here are several stretches to loosen up your arms and shoulders. With your feet flat on the ground and legs spread apart at shoulders width, reach your arms straight up over your head, bringing them closer together, then further apart; then stretch them straight out in front of you, bringing them back and over your head again, alternating between straight up and straight out, back and forth 20 times.

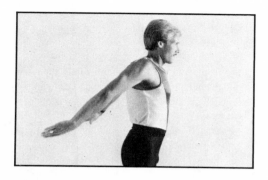

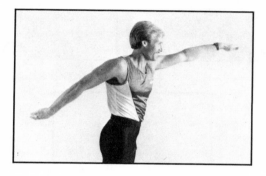

Figure 14a and 14b. *Arm and Back Stretch.* Pull your arms together straight back, then bring one forward, keeping the other back, then alternate, left arm, right arm, back and forth 20 times.

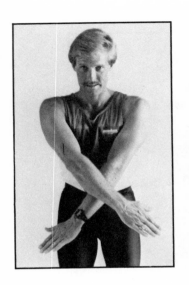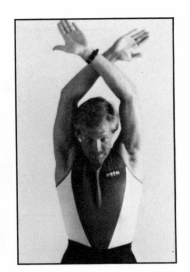

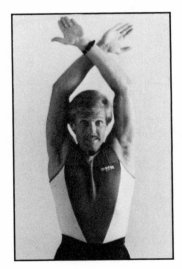

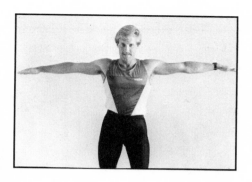

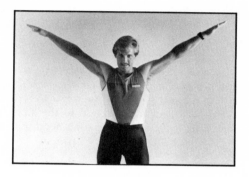

Figure 15a, 15b, 15c, 15d, and 15e. *Arm and Body Stretch.* Begin with your arms at your side, then crisscross your arms in front of you, slowly, then pull them apart and bring them up over your head, criss crossing them above, then bring back down, criss crossing them below, and so on for 25 repetitions.

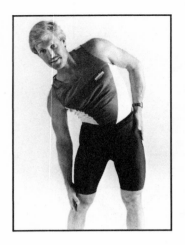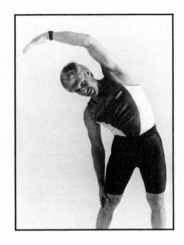

Figure 16a and 16b. *Body Stretch.* To stretch your body, place your right hand on your right thing and stretch your torso to the right, then bring your left arm up and over your head to add to the stretch. Switch to the other side, bringing your right arm over your head and stretch your left arm down your leg. Repeat back and forth 15 times.

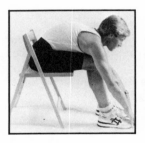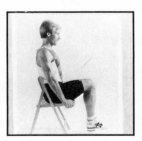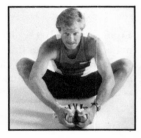

Figure 17. *Sitting Toe Touch.* With your feet flat on the ground, stretch down and touch your toes. Instead of stretching your legs, this one will stretch your back and arms.

Figure 18. *Leg Lift.* Sitting on the chair and grabbing the seat with your hands, lift your legs straight up, keep your feet together and legs bent. Hold the lift for 10 seconds, then place feet on ground. Repeat 15 times.

Figure 19. *Inner Leg Stretch.* Sitting flat on the floor, reach forward and grab your feet with both hands, legs outside of your arms, and stretch your torso as far forward as possible. Hold for 15 seconds, then relax back up. Repeat 10 times.

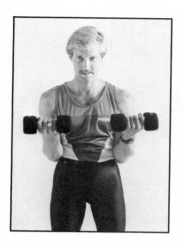 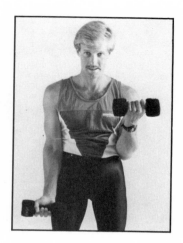

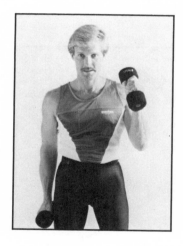

Figure 20a, 20b, and 20c. *Bicep Curls.* Begin with your weights held up as in the first photo. Then lower one while holding the other up. Then switch arms, alternating the weights up and down. A variation on this exercise is shown in the third photo by twisting the weights so that they point forward. The weight system allows you to remove the gel-filled end weights for a lighter system. These terry-cloth lined gel weights can, in turn, be slipped on your wrists or ankles, for an added weight to another part of your body, should you need to adjust any of the weight exercises.

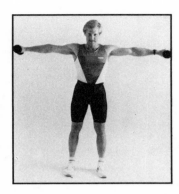

Figure 21. *Tricep Extension.* Begin with the weights at your side, then raise them up together so that your arms are straight out. Hold that position for 10 seconds, then gently lower the weights back down to your side. Repeat 10 times.

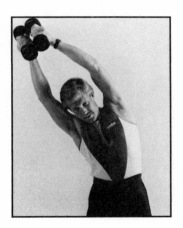

Figure 22. *Torso Sway Extension.* With both weights held over your head, sway your body right, then left, and back right again, back and forth for 20 repetitions. If the system is too heavy, remove the gel-filled weights and just use the lighter bars.

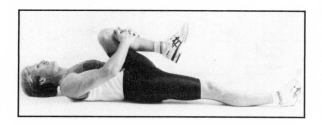

Figure 23. *Leg Pull.* Lying on your back with your right leg extended straight out and flat on the ground (remember to keep your head back against the floor), grab your left leg (bending the knee) and slowly pull it up to your chest as far as you can. Hold it for 5 seconds, then release the leg, and stretch it straight out as you pull your right leg up to your chest. Repeat the movements, left and right, 20 times.

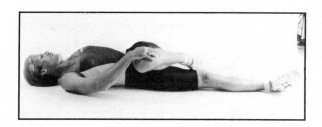

Figure 24. *Hip Stretch.* Lying flat on your back with your right leg extended out, keep your left arm straight out on the floor while you grab your left knee with your right arm and pull it over your right leg so that it stretches your left hip. Hold this stretch for 5 seconds. Do not jerk your leg into this position. Rather, stretch it slowly over. Then release it and do the same stretch with the opposite side. Repeat back and forth 20 times.

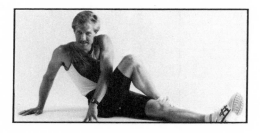

Figure 25. *Hip-Torso Flexor.* Sitting on the ground, with your left leg straight out, place your right foot behind your left leg, while you stretch both hands out toward the ground, twisting your hips and torso. Hold this position for 10 seconds, then reverse. Alternate back and forth 10 times.

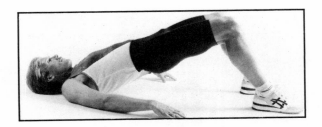

Figure 26. *The Arch.* Lying on the ground, place your arms out flat, at about a 45-degree angle in order to support your body. Push up with your arms and head, arching your back up away from the floor. Hold for 10 seconds, then relax. Repeat 10 times. This will strengthen both your upper arms and shoulders, and your neck.

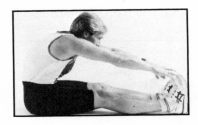

Figure 27. *Hamstring Stretch.* Sitting on the floor, legs straight out, reach forward and touch your toes, keeping your heels forward and toes straight up. This will likely be difficult as most people's hamstrings (the back of your upper legs) are very tight. If necessary, bend your knees temporarily, grab your feet, and then slowly try to straighten your legs. If it is too painful, then work up to it. Hold each stretch for 15 seconds and repeat 10 times.

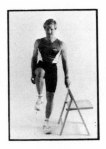

Figure 28. *Leg Lifts.* Positioned next to the chair for support, slowly raise your right leg up, knee bent, and hold for 20 seconds. Then shift to the left leg and repeat the hold. Shift back and forth, for 10 repetitions each leg.

KEYS TO SUCCESSFUL EXERCISE

In all three areas of exercise—stretching, strength, and endurance—the important thing is consistency. Doing something every single day is the best thing you can do for your arthritis. It isn't so important how far you stretch, or how much weight you can lift, or how far you can swim, bike, or run. The important thing is doing them on a daily basis in order to keep your body fit and your joints loose.

Make exercise a normal part of your day—like eating and sleeping. You wouldn't go without eating or sleeping, and you shouldn't go without exercise. Work it into your program first thing in the morning, or during your lunch break, or when you get home from work. Whenever it is, just be consistent so that your mind and body develop a set routine. I strongly recommend stretching and some endurance exercising first thing in the morning in order to get the joints loosened up. Strength training is better (for me anyway) later in the day when my body is in full swing.

What About Pain?

Don't worry about a *little bit* of pain. A little pain is probably good. The Arthritis Foundation suggests that if the pain lasts more than about two hours after the end of an exercise period, you should taper down and rest a little before doing it again. As you become more experienced in exercise and your arthritis, you will "know" your body, and know when to keep going or to stop.

Moderation

The key to a successful exercise program for dealing with arthritis is moderation. The mistake many people make is in assuming that if a little exercise is good then a lot must be great. This is not the case. As much as I love to exercise, and as much as I promote exercise to arthritics, I can't stress enough the importance of being moderate in the amounts of exercise you do. If you have a dream goal of some great athletic feat, you've got to work up to it very slowly. Even though I was already a professional athlete, it took me 16 long months of very gradual increases in exercise to build my mobility, strength, and endurance back up to where I could compete in the Ironman again.

Watch Out for Overtraining

For the majority of athletes in general, overtraining is not a problem because the whole idea of training in the first place is based on progressive overloading, that is, pushing a little harder each time to build your muscles stronger and stronger. It takes a tremendous amount of excessive overloading to reach the point where it becomes overtraining. Most people never reach this level. But for someone with arthritis who is getting into an exercise program, overtraining may more likely be a problem because of the sensitivity of our bodies to *any* overloading, especially a progressive program of overloading.

Symptoms of overtraining in general include:

Increased fatigue even when not exercising
Decreased drive and energy in daily life
Excessive muscle and joint soreness
Weight loss
Decreased resistance to colds and other illnesses
Difficulty in sleeping
Lack of motivation
Arms and legs may feel "heavy"
Resting pulse rate is higher than normal

The general cause of overtraining is, well, overtraining—that is, doing too much of the same thing over and over and over. Physically the cause is glycogen depletion. As discussed in the nutrition chapter, glycogen is the sugarlike substance that fuels the muscles by providing quick energy to make contractions possible. In overtraining, the body never fully recovers its normal stores of glycogen (from eating carbohydrates), and must then begin to consume fats, which are not nearly as efficient a fuel source. The result is a decrease in energy efficiency which causes feelings of fatigue and soreness.

For someone with arthritis, this problem may be intensified because the sensitivity of joints and muscles is usually more than in the non-arthritic body. Thus, you may experience the symptoms of overtraining before the non-arthritic athlete. Muscles may become sore and joints flare up with inflammation due to excessive exercise.

To remedy the problem, I suggest the following:

Take time off from training. Maybe take several days to a week off from your normal routine.

Don't feel guilty about resting. For arthritics, rest is as important as exercise. The right balance is the key, and your body will let you know when it isn't in balance. The symptoms I described above will become noticeable.

After you've rested, change exercises. Do something different. Break up the monotony by trying different sports or exercises.

Keeping a training log, as I suggested earlier, will help you avoid the overtraining problem in the future. Look back to see what you were doing when you began to experience the symptoms of overtraining. You will probably notice a pattern of increased exercise beyond what your body was ready to handle.

Thus, when you do resume exercising, go back to the pre-overtraining levels until you feel strong enough to work your way back up to higher levels, always being sensitive to your body's feedback.

The important thing to remember is that there is a fine line between exercising the right amount to keep your body strong and flexible, and exercising too much so that you are straining your body beyond its capacity to recover. You will discover this point soon enough by listening to your body as it gives you clues through pain and fatigue. I can't tell you where that point is since every body is different. You must discover it on your own, as you push yourself in your exercise program.

SELF-MASSAGE

In recent years, attention has been focused on the use of massage for arthritis sufferers to temporarily relieve sore muscles and stiff joints. A properly trained massage therapist can work wonders with a battered body. Unfortunately, you get what you pay for, and good massage therapists are not exempt from this rule. They can charge anywhere from $25 for a half-hour, half-body massage session to $75 for a full one-hour, full-body massage session. Who can afford a good massage three or four days a week? The solution is self-massage.

The Benefits of Self-massage

While it is advisable to consult a massage therapist first regarding your needs and specific problems, self-massage can give you continuous benefits without extraneous expense.

Self-massage helps you learn about your own body—its aches and pains, tender points, strong and weak spots, and pain tolerance. The more you know about your body, the better able you are to take care of it.

It is convenient and expedient to be able to work on yourself, rather than driving to a clinic for a weekly massage.

Self-massage protects against injury by keeping muscles, ligaments, tendons, and joints loose.

Self-massage acts like biofeedback. Your hands are the biofeedback instrument that your brain monitors. Massage will tell you what state your body is in.

Perhaps most importantly, self-massage is very relaxing. It reduces tension and anxiety and relieves stress. In short, massage feels good. Admittedly, it feels best when someone else massages you, but even working on yourself produces good results.

How to Self-massage

There are almost as many types of massage therapies as there are massage therapists using them. Everyone has his or her own particular, individual method of doing massage. As you work on yourself, you may develop your own special technique that produces the best results for you.

SWEDISH STYLE. This is the type of massage you may have received from a friend who rubbed your back and shoulders. It feels good, is somewhat relaxing, but doesn't really help to alleviate true muscular and joint problems. It is done by applying just enough pressure to make you feel good without any discomfort at all. It should be done with both hands making long sweeping motions in the lengthwise direction of the muscles and, if possible, always toward the heart for improved circulation.

PÉTRISSAGE. This is the kneading of a muscle, almost as if it were a loaf of bread. Cup your hands around the muscle and squeeze it, continuously, on and off, with both hands. The amount of pressure should be enough to really work the muscle so that it feels a little uncomfortable and possibly even a little painful. Another way is to start at the ends of the muscle and work in. If it were the quadriceps, for example, you might start with the palms of your hands up just below your hips and push slowly down toward the muscle's insertion at the knee. You should follow the path of the bone. Most muscles run parallel to bones, so this is a good way to massage them.

ACUPRESSURE.   The third method is taken from the ancient Oriental practice of acupuncture. Acupressure works by pushing down on specific pressure points in the body to relieve muscle tension and pain. For instance, one of the classic pressure points is found between the thumb and forefinger, right behind the major tendon running through this area. Applying pressure here is reported to help relieve headaches, cramps, and nausea.

Dos and Don'ts of Self-massage

1.   Use massage oil or lotions for better motion over the muscles.

2.   Massage after every workout, if possible.

3.   You can even massage your own back by lying on tennis balls and moving around, letting them stay in one place for a few seconds each.

4.   Massage either the length of the muscle or massage it at a 90-degree angle.

5.   Whenever possible, massage toward the heart. This allows the circulation to pump out more quickly the impurities in the system.

6.   Don't massage a muscle or tendon that you think might be injured. If there is swelling or extreme pain, see your doctor or professional therapist.

7.   Don't massage too deep in the style of rolfing (named after Ida Rolf), which is not massage but a tearing apart of the muscle groups.

8. Find a comfortable position on the floor, in a chair, on a couch, or on a bed, and try to relax the body as much as possible.

9. To prevent fatigue in your hands, use your arms and body to apply pressure.

10. Beware of "therapeutic touch" techniques which are based on the concept that the body has an energy field that extends beyond the skin. The "therapeutic touch" therapist "massages" this energy field to "smooth out" aches and pains. Claims are made that this works without even touching the patient. There is no scientific evidence that this works.

Massage is both an art and a science. It requires some knowledge of anatomy and physiology of the muscular and circulatory system and also the ability to apply that knowledge to the healing of the human body, either someone else's or your own.

WATER EXERCISES

Many arthritis sufferers have been doing water workouts for years to get their exercise and relieve arthritis pain at the same time—activities such as water aerobics, jacuzzi gymnastics, and shower stretches. Exercising in the water works one of two ways:

1. Warm water acts to increase circulation and loosen stiff joints.

2. Water itself, when a body is submerged in it, has the effect of attenuating the "heavy" effects of gravity. You are practically weightless in water, so this is a great place to do exercises that are almost stress-free on the joints.

WATER AEROBICS. In addition to lap-swimming, of course, many public and private pools, health clubs, and

YMCAs hold daily water aerobics classes for people of all ages, but they often gear them to pregnant women and people with arthritis. Running in place, stretching, twisting, kicking, and so on are all great joint looseners, and there is almost no way you can hurt yourself.

JACUZZI GYMNASTICS. If you don't have a pool handy, a jacuzzi may be even better because the water is hotter, making it even easier for you to stretch your muscles and increase your range of motion. In your jacuzzi you can, for instance, push your fingers and hands against the side wall, stretching them back from your wrist. You can place your leg on one of the stairs with the other leg on the floor, and stretch to touch your toes on the foot on the stair. You can loosen your knees by pulling your foot back up against the back of your leg, and so on. Be creative. Nothing feels better for arthritis than a good hot tub. Enjoy the moment but put it to good use while you're in there.

SHOWER STRETCHES. If you don't have a pool or jacuzzi, a great way to start the morning or end the day is a good hot shower where you take an extra couple of minutes to do a number of stretches. Take advantage of the hot water to keep those joints loose.

All in all I can't say enough about the benefits of exercise for health in general and arthritis in particular. For me exercise was the vehicle that drove me to freedom from anxiety and near-freedom from pain. I don't claim that exercise is a panacea for arthritis, but if you want to meet the physical challenge head-on, there is no better arena than that of physical exercise.

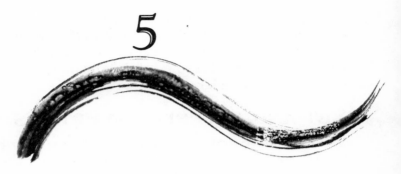

CHAPTER 5

Arthritis and Nutrition

"One should eat to live, not live to eat."

—BENJAMIN FRANKLIN

Like many arthritics, I went through a period where I tried virtually every "remedy" that I could get my hands on. Since the time I first began looking into ways to relieve my arthritis symptoms there was always one strategy staring me in the face wherever I went—nutrition. Bookstores and library shelves are filled with books on diet and nutrition in general, and specialized diets for people with sundry disorders—arthritis included. Fish oils, amino acids, vitamins, prostaglandins, the omega-3 fatty acids, EPA, ALA, DHA (explained below), calcium, B complex, and so on—all have claimants who swear the right dosages or combinations thereof will relieve arthritis symptoms. In this chapter I'd like to address the issue of arthritis and nutrition and tell you about some of the claims for the effectiveness of a specialized diet, review what doctors and scientists offer us in the way of evidence for some of these claims, and discuss the benefits of a well-balanced diet.

DIET AND ARTHRITIS SYMPTOMS

Can diet relieve arthritis symptoms? In two words, no and yes. *No*, specialized nutrition and miracle diets do not work in relieving arthritis symptoms. But having made that blanket statement, let me qualify it by explaining that for me, and within the scientific community, there is no evidence that nutrition alone can relieve arthritis symptoms.

I've tried virtually every nutritional program there is and have personally experienced no relief of symptoms due strictly to the diet. But let me also note that in general I eat a well-balanced, healthy diet. My exercise program demands that I eat plenty of carbohydrates, high fiber, and starchy foods. I stay away from fats, sugars, high sodium, and alcohol. This is not a specialized arthritis diet. It is a normal, healthy diet that all doctors recommend for all their patients to promote good health. I have experienced much relief from my arthritis symptoms, but this is likely due to a combination of factors, including a balanced diet, exercise, anti-inflammatory medication, and a positive mental attitude. So to the extent that arthritis symptoms are affected by general health, and general health is improved by a balanced, proper diet, then *yes*, nutrition can make a difference.

Scientific Evidence

Scientifically, there is no data that supports any of the nutritional claims for arthritis relief; that is, a specific diet alone has not been proven to be an effective arthritis relief measure. By scientifically I mean controlled experiments where one group of arthritis sufferers eats a specialized diet for an extended period of time—the experimental group—and another group of arthritis sufferers eats a different diet, a diet without the test foods, for an extended period of time—the control group. These groups are carefully selected to make sure that all arthritis sufferers have the same type of arthritis, are of a similar age, contain an equal number of men and women, and so on. This is to control for other variables that might affect the arthritis symptoms. Then the scientists must have a way of measuring improvement—such as a decrease in inflammation and pain—and then compare the two groups to see if there is a significant difference between the two. Thus far, there have been no successful experiments supporting any claims that specialized nutrition can relieve arthritis symptoms.

Other Evidence

Is scientific evidence the only evidence to consider? Well, again, I must answer yes and no. *Yes*, scientific evidence is the only evidence to consider if you want to make generalized claims about the benefits of nutrition for relieving arthritis symptoms. We must have controlled experimental data to draw scientific conclusions. *No*, scientific evidence is not the only evidence to consider if you want to make specific claims that fish oils (for example) helped an individual feel better—we can't dispute such personal claims. Perhaps it really did help. Optimizing arthritis relief means trying different things to see what works for you.

For myself, I tried virtually everything, and absolutely nothing worked. So I've drawn my conclusions and I agree with the scientists. Science has not proven that such claims are false. Science has only concluded that they are not true. The difference is in the nature of evidence. Thus far, under controlled conditions, there is no evidence that specified diets work to cure or alleviate arthritis. On the other hand, scientific evidence cannot prove that they don't work for individuals. What works for you may not work for an experimental group, and vice versa. In other words, a certain diet may very well work for you, and if it does, who cares that it didn't work for the experimental group?

It should be noted here that even the conservative Arthritis Foundation recognizes that there are some linkages between diet and certain forms of arthritis. Gout, osteoporosis, and Reiter's syndrome have connections to diet, but these are causal connections, not curative or relief ones. In other words, the diet causes or worsens the disease; it doesn't cure or relieve symptoms.

GOUT.   Foods high in purines (purines are a white, crystalline compound derived from uric acid) such as wine, anchovies, beer, gravies, and liver, can worsen the symptoms of gout. They do this because gout decreases your body's ability to get rid of purines, and an excessive amount of purine in your body can increase the levels of uric acid in the blood and thus increase the chance of an attack of gout, which is caused by a buildup of uric acid crystals in the joints. Therefore, it is recommended that people with gout avoid these types of food.

OSTEOPOROSIS.   Calcium is one of the primary ingredients in making your bones strong. Osteoporosis causes the bones to lose their strength and become more brittle. Diets high in alcohol (more than two drinks a day) and low in calcium (less than 500 milligrams a day) increase the probability of getting this form of arthritis. But once you've got it, taking calcium by itself will not cure or relieve symptoms. For other reasons, however (such as overall bone strength), it is important to maintain a normal amount of calcium in your diet. Women especially may need approximately 1000 to 1500 milligrams a day.

REITER'S SYNDROME.   It has been discovered that water or food poisoning caused by salmonella or other kinds of bacteria may trigger the onset of Reiter's syndrome.

CLAIMS AND UNPROVEN DIETS

The following is a list of some of the foods and supplements that people have claimed have a curative agent or relieving potential. At this point in time, no scientific evidence exists for their specific ability to alleviate arthritis symptoms:

ALA (Alpha Linolenic Acid)
Alfalfa
Arachidonic acid
Black walnuts
Copper
Copper salts
Dairy products
DHA (Docosahexaenoic Acid)
EPA (Eicosapentaenoic Acid)
Fiber
Fish oils
GLA (Gamma Linolenic Acid)
Immune power diet
Linoleic acid
No meats/preservatives diet
No nightshades diet
Omega-3 fatty acids
Plant oils
Prostaglandins
Sodium nitrates
Vinegar and honey
Vitamin B complex
Vitamin C
Zinc

Arthritis diet book claims are bold. "Arthritis relief is within your power. All you have to do is make a personal commitment to follow the diet revealed in this book," reads the opening sentence of one recent publication. "Calcium, along with the vitamin B complex and vitamins C and E have been found particularly important for the prevention and relief of arthritis and rheumatism," says another recent author, quoting an older work on arthritis.

Fish and Fish Oil

The claims usually center around eating fish and fish oils, an idea that came from studies showing that Eskimos in Greenland and Alaska show virtually no signs of arthritis, and they also consume large amounts of fish. Is there a direct connection? Most likely not. Recent research has revealed that in the late Middle Ages almost no one had arthritis, no matter where they lived. Then the disease spread throughout Europe and America, possibly as a virus through ticks carried by certain species of deer, which would jump from the deer onto people. The causal chain from the virus to arthritis is a long and complex one and needn't concern us here. Perhaps Eskimos have simply never been exposed to the virus.

The diet–arthritis-relief connection is as follows: Inflammation is linked to certain amounts and types of prostaglandins, chemicals naturally produced by the body. The supposed "beneficial" prostaglandins are made from a fatty acid called eicosapentaenoic acid, or EPA, that is found in marine plants and fish. EPA is one of the three fatty acids in the much-touted omega-3 fatty acids that many arthritis diet books claim relieve symptoms. The other two are alpha linolenic acid (ALA) and docosahexaenoic acid (DHA). How does this work? ALA is one of the building blocks of EPA, and DHA is produced from EPA, and all three are found in algae, plankton, and fish. Since EPA is linked to the "beneficial" prostaglandins that are supposed to help reduce inflammation, by logical inference one should eat such fish as anchovy, cod, flounder, herring, halibut, mackerel, sardines, salmon, snapper, trout, tuna, and so on, in order to relieve arthritis symptoms.

At this time there is no strong scientific evidence to support this connection other than a report in the *Journal of Rheumatology* that patients receiving 18 grams of fish oil daily with their arthritis medication reported significant relief from joint tenderness as well as improved grip ability. However, since the medical estabishment does recommend eating more fish for various other reasons such as protection against heart disease and cancer, a more fish-based diet might not be such a bad idea.

The Nightshade/Food Allergy Question

According to Dr. Norman Childers, a former horticulture professor at Rutgers University, certain chemical substances in the nightshade family of plants (tomatoes, white potatoes, eggplant, and garden peppers) cause a toxic reaction in the body that triggers inflammation and pain. In his book *The Nightshades and Health,* Dr. Childers and his coauthor Gerard Russo state that members of the nightshade family contain a substance called solanine, which destroys one of the enzymes that helps keep our muscles flexible. They note that livestock that eat the leaves of these plants get calcification in their soft tissues. They conclude that the active ingredient of vitamin D, which they claim is known to cause arthritis, is in these plants.

The no-nightshade diet requires giving up everything that contains potatoes, tomatoes, and so forth, such as clam chowder, baked beans, barbecued chicken (tomatoes in the sauce), and ketchup, not to mention avoiding all the foods that contain derivatives of potatoes and tomatoes. Childers and Russo claim that of 1000 people who followed this diet, 70 percent said they experienced some relief.

Once again, the anecdotal evidence from individuals, and non-replicated studies such as the one just cited, may lead you to give it a try, and if it works, then great. But I wouldn't make the assumption that this is a guarantee of arthritis relief.

In addition, there are some who maintain that other foods, such as dairy products, wheat, and especially citrus fruits, are implicated in arthritis inflammation and pain. These individuals suggest that you eliminate all dairy products, wheat, and citrus fruits, and then reintroduce them one at a time to see if your arthritis symptoms get worse. This way you are conducting an experiment on yourself by controlling the effects of each food type. The assertions center around the concept of food allergies—that is, these foods cause an allergic reaction in your body, thus increasing inflammation in the joints.

The field of food allergies, however, is highly controversial in general, and especially so in its purported connection to arthritis. Medical researchers have recently become extremely leery of food allergy testing procedures, which are conducted in test tubes outside the body and seldom resemble the complex chemical reactions going on inside the body. For example, several years ago Michael became involved with a food allergy laboratory that tested him for food allergies and discovered he was allergic to wheat and dairy products. As he systematically eliminated all foods containing wheat or dairy products, or their derivatives, he was losing weight and growing weak and irritable. Skeptical of the whole procedure, Michael subsequently submitted several blood samples from himself, taken at the same time, but told the laboratory they were from different people. Sure enough, each one of the same blood samples showed radically different food allergies, thus negating the entire testing procedure!

As we've seen thus far, there are many claims but few substantiated findings. But as part of our goal to *optimize* your chances of arthritis relief, the best way to find out if something works is to try it yourself. You know your body better than anyone else.

Personal Experimentation

If I seem a little hard on some of the people who make these spectacular claims about arthritis relief from diet, it is because I've gone through most of these programs and had some pretty wild experiences. For example, I remember when I first got home out of the hospital I headed straight for a health food store. I hobbled into the store, barely able to walk and hurting like you wouldn't believe. I went to the book section to see if they had anything on arthritis. Sure enough! There they were. Lots of books about how to cure arthritis with diet, or how natural herbs will relieve arthritis pain, and so on. I purchased several, read them carefully, and then returned to the market to buy all the stuff I needed to get well.

One of the books told me I should drink buckthorn root tea. Buckthorn root is supposed to be an anti-inflammatory, so for weeks I drank this rancid-tasting stuff, thinking that any time now I'd get better. I didn't.

Then I tried a diet of nothing but wheatgrass. After that it was tofu, because another book said that if you just eat tofu, and nothing but tofu, the arthritis pain will go away. Already too skinny from losing so much weight in the hospital, I was losing muscle mass because I was slowly starving myself, and my body began to deteriorate.

For months I tried out all these extreme remedies. Nothing worked. I even tried enemas because another book said that the cause of arthritis pain is impurities in the joints and body. The way to get rid of these toxins was to cleanse the body in two ways: eat whole foods and take enemas, three and four times a day!

This personal experimentation went on for four or five

months until I finally gave up and decided that these drastic, unbalanced diets for relieving arthritis were not helping my body. But if you think about it, recall the first time you experienced arthritis symptoms. Were you eating any differently? Did you change your diet and then get arthritis? I suspect not (with the exception of gout, osteoporosis, or Reiter's syndrome). And since you've had arthritis, have you noticed any consistent relief of symptoms linked to any specific food groups? (I say *consistent* in order to control for the normal ups and downs of arthritis symptoms, as well as for the possibility of symptom remission.) I also suspect not. If these "miracle" diets really worked don't you think the medical community would have published the amazing findings by now? They haven't. And if these "miracle" diets really worked, don't you think millions of arthritis sufferers would now be throwing away their pain killers and anti-inflammatory drugs? They aren't. With the wide variety of arthritis diseases and symptoms, does it make sense that one particular type of diet would be able to relieve symptoms for most or all of them? It doesn't. Finally, the fact that there is such a variety of diets touted as effective in treating arthritis symptoms tells us that it is likely that there is nothing to them.

Because the causes of arthritis are not known, and because there are so many kinds of arthritis, the effects of varied diets on different individuals might not show up in controlled experiments. Therefore, there is something you can do with your nutrition that may make a difference. It has nothing to do with miracle cures. It is just plain old sound nutritional advice.

THE NUTRITION–HEALTH CONNECTION

Whether or not any of these claims are absolutely true (for everyone) or relatively true (for specific individuals), a well-balanced, healthy diet certainly can't hurt, and most likely will help—indirectly. By indirectly I mean the degree of symptom severity or symptom relief is certainly correlated with overall health. This is the positive side of the nutrition–arthritis connection. The healthier you are, the less likely arthritis symptoms will bother you. But if you are overweight, out of shape, have poor circulation, and so on, then of course your symptoms will bother you more. Why? Because being the proper weight keeps those extra pounds (and stress) off your joints, good circulation helps keep joints cleansed and better lubricated, and being in good physical shape makes your muscles stronger and looser for easier joint movement.

It has been scientifically proven that nutrition is directly related to health. So from nutrition to health, and from health to arthritis, there is a causal relationship, albeit indirect. An obvious example is weight. The heavier you are (over your normal body weight as determined by your height, sex, and body type) the more stress there will be on your bones, joints, ligaments, tendons, and muscles. Weight is directly related to nutrition. Eating right and exercising helps you maintain a normal weight, thus decreasing the strain on your body. This may not only prevent further spread of arthritic symptoms, but likely even decrease the amount of inflammation.

In addition, many adults with arthritis who are overweight and don't exercise also have other physical problems such as high blood pressure and heart disease. Good nutrition will positively affect other physical systems, which of course, will make you feel better abut yourself so that the mental game will change the physical game. (More on this in the second half of the book.)

A HEALTHY, BALANCED DIET

The Arthritis Foundation recommends the following seven guidelines leading toward a healthier nutrition program:

1. Eat a variety foods
2. Maintain ideal weight
3. Avoid too much fat and cholesterol
4. Avoid too much sugar
5. Eat foods with enough starch and fiber
6. Avoid too much sodium
7. If you drink alcohol, drink in moderation

But please keep in mind that these are not measures that will relieve arthritis symptoms directly. A balanced diet promotes overall better health, which will likely affect arthritis symptoms because being healthy makes you feel better.

Maximize, Optimize, Minimize

The standard American diet consists of these proportions: carbohydrates—40 percent, proteins—15 percent, and fats—45 percent.

Building a healthy nutritional program is really quite straightforward and simple: maximize carbohydrates, optimize proteins, and minimize fats. I recommend the following percentages: carbohydrates—60 percent, proteins—10 percent, and fats—20 percent. Such a radical reduction in fats from 45 percent to 20 percent perhaps might best be done in stages to avoid the physical cravings that may follow. In general, however, I've found that even in actively trying to eat *no* fats whatsoever, it is unavoidable that I end up consuming a minimum of 10 percent anyway. So my recommendation is to taper off slowly and then try to absolutely minimize fats, since they will come in so many hidden sources anyway, such as sauces, salad dressings, and cooking oils.

The sort of foods that make up the above categories are most commonly the following:

Carbohydrates:
Cereals
Fruits (fresh, dry, or in juice form)
Vegetables (raw or steamed)
Rice
Potatoes
Grains (breads, pancakes)

Proteins:
Meats (poultry, fish, shellfish, veal, beef, duck, pork, lamb)
Legumes (beans, peas, lentils)
Nuts and seeds
Dairy products (milk, cheese, yogurt, cottage cheese—
nonfat or lowfat whenever possible)

Fats:
Oil
Butter
Margarine
Mayonnaise
Ice cream

Carbohydrates

To determine the correct amounts of the right type of foods
you must understand the physiology of the human body.
Physiologists have traced the sequence of energy transfer
as follows: *food—glycogen—glucose—blood—muscle*. When a
muscle can't get the glucose (a type of sugar) it needs from
the blood, it uses its own store of glycogen (a storage carbohydrate converted from sugar and carbohydrate foods)
faster. This is why it is better to eat small meals several
times throughout the day, rather than one or two huge meals.

The primary fuel source for energy (to increase glycogen stores) is carbohydrates. There are two types of carbohydrates—simple and complex. Simple carbohydrates are found in sugar and may provide an immediate but temporary source of energy to fuel the body—in other words, it pumps glucose into the blood stream, but since it runs out quickly the muscles then begin to use the body's store of glycogen. Complex carbohydrates are found in foods such as grains, cereals, vegetables, fruits, green leafy vegetables, pasta, whole-grain breads, and potatoes. For a healthy diet it is best to maximize complex carbohydrates. Essentially they can do no harm, and since they are the primary source of energy, it is best to eat complex carbohydrates regularly throughout the day.

The connection to arthritis is again an indirect one. A steady flow of energy throughout the day will make you stronger, healthier, and feel better overall, making it easier to move and deal with pain.

Proteins

Little of the energy you use throughout a day comes from protein sources, and may amount to less than four percent. However, protein is essential in the construction of enzymes, the catalysts involved in all cellular metabolic processes, as well as the structural components of cells. In other words, there are two types of proteins: structural proteins (the material of cells), and enzymes (the function of cells). Proteins themselves are made of amino acids, which have been called the building blocks of life. There are 20 amino acids in nature, 19 of which are contained in various foods. They are divided into two groups: essential and nonessential. Essential amino acids are necessary for growth and development, and come from foods. Nonessential amino acids are produced by the body.

Proteins are divided into complete and incomplete. Complete proteins contain all the essential amino acids, while incomplete proteins are missing one or more amino acids. Complete proteins are included in the list of foods above. Complete proteins are found in meat, poultry, fish, and dairy products. Incomplete proteins include grains, vegetables, and nuts. An omnivorous diet containing both animal and plant foods will provide all essential amino acids. Vegetarians must combine incomplete proteins in order to provide all the essential amino acids. For protein synthesis to occur, all the essential amino acids must be present. The "Recommended Daily Allowance" (RDA) figure for protein, for a 150-pound individual, is 54 grams a day. This is easily met by a diet containing the protein percentage I've recommended above.

Fats

The metabolism of fats can also be a vital source of energy, especially if your body is short of complex carbohydrates. Fats, however, require more oxygen to utilize as a fuel source, so they are not as efficient. If fats can be a source of energy, then what type of fats should you eat? If you are aiming for a 10 percent daily intake of fat, then one tablespoon of olive oil, vegetable oil (safflower, corn, or sesame), margarine, or mayonnaise is recommended a day. Fats are organized into two categories: saturated and unsaturated (including polyunsaturated and monosaturated). Saturated fat comes mainly from animal sources and is in a solid form at room temperature. Unsaturated fat is liquid at room temperature and is generally found in plant foods. It is the saturated fats that have been linked with increased cholesterol levels in the blood, itself linked to heart disease. Whenever possible, use polyunsaturated fats instead of saturated fats. In other words, replace butter with corn and soy oil, or derivative margarines. The American Heart Association suggests eating the "friendly" fats found in salmon and mackerel, and the "essential" fats that occur in such foods as oatmeal, corn, and brown rice. The American diet and most American restaurant foods are so rich in fat that even if you think you are avoiding fats altogether you are probably getting more than the daily allotment.

Sodium and Salt

In addition to eating a healthy, balanced diet, there are other factors to consider in diet and nutrition. As a result of certain anti-inflammatory medications many arthritics have high blood pressure and either diarrhea or constipation. Therefore, consuming complex carbohydrates in the form of fiber foods—whole-grain breads, cereal, popcorn, vegetables, fruits, and so on—can be good not only for energy, but to also keep your bowel movements regular. Furthermore, if you have high blood pressure it may be helpful to limit the amount of sodium/salt you consume a day. Also, certain arthritis drugs, such as corticosteroids, may cause the body to retain higher than normal amounts of sodium, and some people have argued that excess sodium may increase arthritis pain, though this has yet to be proven.

Alcohol

Consuming beer, wine, and hard liquor is tempting as a mode to deal with pain, both physically and psychologically. But while it isn't necessary you eliminate alcohol entirely from your diet, keeping it at a minimum is certainly sound advice. In addition to increasing weight (because of the extra sugar), alcohol may intefere with the medication you are taking for arthritis. Moreover, alcohol may cause a deterioration of the stomach lining, which, in conjunction with certain drugs (like the anti-inflammatory nonsteroidals) may cause excessive damage to the stomach. The following drugs are not recommended in conjunction with alcohol by the Arthritis Foundation:

Generic Name	Some Brand Names
Acetaminophen	Anacin-3, Datril, Panodol, Tylenol
Allopurinol	Lopurin, Zyloprim
Colchicine	Colchicine
Diflunisal	Dolobid
Fenoprofen	Nalfon
Ibuprofen	Advil, Medipren, Motrin, Nuprin
Indomethacin	Indocin
Ketoprofen	Orudis
Meclofenamate	Meclomen
Naproxen	Naprosyn
Phenylbutazone	Azolid, Butazolidin
Piroxicam	Feldene
Probenecid	Benemid, SK-Probenecid
Salicylate (Aspirin)	Anacin, Bayer, Bufferin, Zorprin
Sulfinpyrazone	Anturane
Sulindac	Clinoril
Tolmetin	Tolectin

Caffeine and Sugar

Although I'm certainly not suggesting that you eliminate all caffeine and sugar, an excess of these can cause irritability and hyperactivity, neither of which help the arthritis sufferer. Coffee is one of my vices, but I've had to keep the consumption of it to a minimum.

THE NUTRITION–MENTAL CHALLENGE CONNECTION

In conclusion, there is a connection between nutrition and arthritis. That linkage is the indirect one I spoke of earlier: Proper nutrition leads to good health; good health leads to a stronger, more efficient body; a stronger, more efficient body leads to a positive mental attitude; and a positive mental attitude can help you deal with your arthritis in a way that can allow you to lead a total and involved life again. It is this mental game to which I now turn in the subsequent chapters.

The
Mental
Challenge

"The most glorious moments in your life are not the so-called days of success, but rather those days when out of dejection and despair you feel rise in you a challenge to life, and the promise of future accomplishments."

—GUSTAVE FLAUBERT

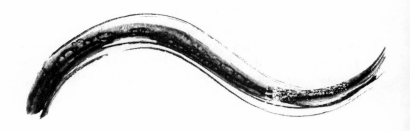

Now that we've reviewed the medical aspects of arthritis, and examined the effects of exercise and nutrition on arthritis symptoms—the *physical challenge*—it is time to give that challenge a direction down a path not previously traveled—the *mental challenge*. Regardless of what your new goals may be—whether it's a physical, psychological, intellectual, or spiritual end you seek—there are certain principles that apply to all who desire to better themselves. The following five chapters are the principles of the *mental challenge* of psyching yourself into greater levels of achievement. Since there is no absolute outside authority to tell us what we should achieve, we must look within to discover those desires. What is right for one person may not be for another. Every individual's goals will be different, but *how* to achieve those goals can be understood within these five chapters which cover: taking up the new challenge (chapter 6), setting goals (chapter 7), achieving goals (chapter 8), dealing with failure (chapter 9), and integrating the physical and mental challenge (chapter 10). The *mental challenge* is the engine that drives you to overcome the *physical challenge*. Integrating these two will help you lead a more balanced lifestyle so that you may become a participant again.

6

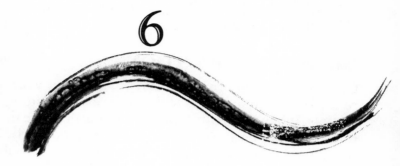

Back to Square One: Taking Up the New Challenge

"What on earth would a man do with himself if something did not stand in his way?"

—H.G. WELLS

Having arthritis has been one long learning experience for me—like starting life over again. When you get arthritis you really don't know what's going on. You don't know what's happening to you. I knew this was not the type of pain I had experienced from bike racing or triathlons. This was something different. To be honest, I was in shock. I couldn't imagine myself with arthritis. Because of this shock I think we all experience, we have to go back to the basics, back to the beginning of understanding ourselves—what I call going *back to square one.*

IMPORTANT QUESTIONS

Going back to square one means reassessing your situation, relearning basic physical skills, and re-establishing your potentials. When I initially entered the hospital, the first thing I realized was that I wasn't going to get well quickly. I knew it was going to be a long road, a long journey of rehabilitation. At that moment I asked myself a series of very important questions. What I call the *who, what, where, when,* and *why* questions: *Who do I want to be? What do I want to do? Where do I want to go? When will I get there?* And *Why do I want to be me?* We will examine each of these questions from a general perspective, followed by some practical, real-world examples, and finally some square one principles to help you take up the challenge of arthritis.

Who Do I Want to Be?

Because *who* you are is a reasonably important matter in your life, the answer to this question should be thought out carefully. It sets the direction for the other four questions. With me, for example, I decided that I wanted to be a competitor again, and that I wanted to be the best I could be. I wanted to "go for it." So I planted that seed as my long-range goal, with a time limit on how long it would take.

Since the answer to this question sets the pace for the others, I would offer one general piece of advice in thinking about your answer: *Don't sell yourself short.* Until you've tried all the options, no one knows, neither you nor your doctor, just *who* you are capable of being. The only way to find out is by trying. I didn't have to say that I wanted to be a competitor again. I could have just said I wanted to walk again, and I would have accomplished that but no more. I know when you are lying there and can hardly even move, setting some crazy goal in the distant future of who you would like to be may seem absurd, but that is what will motivate you through the whole step-by-step process of recovery.

What Do I Want to Do?

Who you want to be will then give you a sense for *what* you want to do. For me, "I want to be a competitor" meant "I want to do the Ironman." There were, of course, a hundred steps in between, but those hundred steps led to something. I discovered you don't go from *A* to *Z*, you go from *A* to *B* to *C* to *D*, and so on.

With each step you get stronger and can push yourself a little harder. Hope is tied to progress. Progress is tied to work. And work is tied to continuity—sticking with *what* you want to do until you get it. From the time when I was lying in bed unable to move—the time I decided *what* I wanted to do—to when I could run again was over 10 months. It was a long, slow process. But once you've gotten there, it doesn't seem so long.

So in a sense, the answer to this question is also very important because it sets the direction for *where* you want to go from square one.

Where Do I Want to Go?

This question may be answered two different ways. In a general sense you may want to answer the question as I did. When I asked myself, "Where do I want to go?," I answered, "As far as I can." So the first step is to affirm to yourself that you are worthy of doing all that you are capable of doing—of going as far as you can go.

But as far as you can go, where? *Where* implies a direction. If you don't know where you are going, then any road will take you there. So the second step is to pick a road down which to travel. Once you've answered the *who* and *what* questions, the *where* answer should naturally follow. For example, if *who* you want to be is a normal, active, reasonably pain-free person, and *what* you want to do is certain activities, then *where* you go, specifically, are to the places and people who will help you get there. You go to books, magazines, journals, and lectures to learn about arthritis. You go to doctors and researchers to get expert advice. You go to therapists to help you rehabilitate. You go to the Arthritis Foundation to learn about the latest research in arthritis. You participate in fund-raising activities to support research in arthritis. You go to support groups to learn how others have become normal, active, and reasonably pain-free.

In other words, affirm that you want to go as far as you can, then get specific on exactly where you want to go.

When Will I Get There?

When you will get there, of course, depends on the type of arthritis you've got, the severity of the condition, and how motivated you are to rehabilitate. While in my case being an athlete before might have helped me get to where I wanted to go, on another level it didn't help me get there sooner, because I was starting completely over. I knew I could push myself, but I didn't know how far or how hard. And in some cases, this caused problems because I pushed myself too hard, as I was used to expecting more out of my body.

The problem with such long-range aspirations, of course, is that it's a long row to hoe. You don't just get out of bed and start running. I had to get out of bed into a wheelchair, and then use crutches, and then a walker. My muscles were totally atrophied, I had lost 45 pounds, and I was so weak I could hardly stand up. I needed help in just getting out of bed and moving at all. I had to draw on every resource that I had, both mentally and physically.

So, first and foremost, you've got to work closely with your doctor or therapist who will show you what steps to take, and how soon it is reasonable to take them. Yet, you can't depend on the therapist to push you or hold you back. Only you know how you feel, so you've got to listen to your body.

Why Do I Want to Be Me?

This question is a little deeper than the others, because it underlies the other four. It is, in a sense, the engine that drives you to pursue answers to *who, what, where,* and *when.* Answering the *why* question means knowing for what purpose you are trying to answer those questions, and once you've answered them, keeping you on track to obtain those answers. For me, the answer to the question *Why do I want to be me?* is: because I want to know in the end that I was able to get all that I could out of life and that I would never have to say, "I wonder if I could've . . . ," "I wish I would've . . . ," and so on. Don't be a "wanna be." Be an "I am me" and know why you are.

PRINCIPLES IN ACTION: BEBE GREEN MEETS HER CHALLENGE

One of the best things I did in my rehabilitation process was to get involved with the Arthritis Foundation. Through this organization I have had the opportunity to meet many people who have gone through similar experiences as myself. It was very motivating and inspiring to me to know that others have suffered and survived. And not only survived, but succeeded. One such person is Bebe Green.

Bebe Green was diagnosed with rheumatoid arthritis at the age of 45. In 10 years she has not only come back to be the socially active, dynamic person she was before the arthritis, she has developed a philosophy in life—that of being the server instead of the served—that would not have developed had she not had the challenge of arthritis. Yet for Bebe, now nearly fully recovered after 10 years, the initial challenge came as a complete surprise: "Frankly I was shocked—devastated really. I couldn't believe I had arthritis. It took me awhile just to be able to accept the concept."

Bebe's dismay and disbelief were understandable, considering her arthritis was triggered by the extreme stress of a large kidney stone that had destroyed two-thirds of her kidney. Doctors think that the arthritis might have been caused by the shock and poison from the ordeal. The arthritis struck hard and fast. "I went from being an extremely active person to lying flat out on my bed unable to move. One day I was water-skiing and playing the guitar and piano; the next day I couldn't even move."

Like many of us at the beginning of our challenge, Bebe tried anything and everything to relieve the symptoms— from the proven to the unproven (including Australian mussels). Finally, what worked reasonably well for her was gold saline shots: at first daily, then weekly, then monthly, and finally bi-monthly, until after two years she tapered off completely, most of her symptoms in remission. "It took about three months of the gold injections before I saw any improvement. Between the gold, immunosuppressent drugs, and other steps, it was about three years between first contracting arthritis and leveling off at the level I am at now."

Those "other steps" are not so much curative ones as they are steps for living a full life. And a full life it is that Bebe now leads. In addition to being executive director for the Coachella (California) branch of the Arthritis Foundation, Bebe is social director for the Marriot Rancho Las Palmas Resort, a job that requires her to once again be the active person she was before the arthritis challenge, and to be that person she decided to be when she answered the question *who do I want to be?* with *the same person I was before.*

Is she the same person as before? "I'm not quite as active as I was before getting arthritis, but I have just as much fun, if not more, doing what I can do. I can't play the guitar and piano like I did before, but I still do play and enjoy it. I can't water-ski anymore, but I can sit in the boat, root others on, and have just as much fun as I used to." But make no mistake about it—Bebe Green leads a full, active life, as much as, if not more than, most non-arthritic people I know. How does she do it? Her daily routine offers us all some excellent tips in coping with arthritic pain, protecting joints, and building muscular strength and flexibility. For example:

IN BED.   Every morning before she even gets out of bed Bebe does leg extensions by lying on her back and stretching each leg, extended straight out, up toward the ceiling. Making the movements slowly, this opens up her range of motion so that walking seems easy by comparison. She also does pelvic tilts. Lying flat on your back, you can do these by squeezing the buttock muscles together and tilting the pelvis upward so that the small of your back is pushed flat against the bed. This strengthens not only your lower back and buttocks, but also the abdomen region.

IN THE SHOWER.   When she takes a shower Bebe uses this as another opportunity to loosen up her joints and gain greater flexibility and range of motion. For example, with hot water flowing over her body making the joints warm, Bebe then does a series of stretching moves and isometric exercises that let her start the day fully charged. For example, she pushes her fingers against the wall, stretching them back from the palm of the hand, thus extending the range of motion of her fingers and wrist. Also, bent over at the waist, she stretches her arms up over her head and toward the ceiling, like a ballet move, which works the upper arms and shoulders. With her back to the shower-head and the hot water running over her neck, she rotates her head around in circles, increasing that range of motion. An isometric exercise she does is to push her hands together, arms against the wall, and to move the arms up and down, from the abdomen to the chin. And so forth. You can create your own series of stretches and exercises that are suitable for your particular points of strengths and weaknesses.

IN THE HOT TUB.   Bebe takes advantage of relaxing in the hot tub by using the jets and hot water for yet another opportunity to keep the joints loose. For example, in a hot tub you can do all sorts of stretches, such as stretching the back of your legs by standing in the middle of the hot tub, placing your foot up on the stairs, and stretching to touch your toes. Or, standing in the middle of the hot tub, grab your foot and pull it up against the back of your leg, thus stretching your thighs. Bebe says, "Be creative!"

To give you an example of just how active a woman Bebe is, while we were talking on the phone discussing this book, she was riding a stationary bike during the entire conversation! This is a woman who has a purpose, a goal. She knows *who* she is, *what* she is doing, *where* she is going, *when* she plans to get there, and *why* she is doing it all. Her philosophy, as I mentioned above, is to be a server, not to be served. "I don't want people to think of me as handicapped or disabled. I don't. I know who I am and I just want to be treated like that. I know what I wanted to do when I got arthritis. I wanted to be in the mainstream of life again, not on the sidelines."

But this is no idealistic, denial strategy. Bebe, like all of us, has her moments of pain and doubt. "Sure, it gets depressing occasionally. But I try not to let it get me down." How does she do this? With a strong support structure. "I've got a very supporting family who are always there when I need them. You've got to surround yourself with positive people and things." This challenge has reshaped Bebe's outlook on life. "For me, life counts every day, every minute, but it was always like this for me, even before I got arthritis. All the arthritis did was to heighten the effect."

The Arthritis Foundation theme for 1990 is "Your source of hope and health." Bebe Green is the embodiment of that philosophy. She has turned the challenge of arthritis into an outward philosophy, instead of an inward one. In other words, Bebe doesn't dwell on what she *can't* do, rather she focuses on what she *can* do, especially in the way of helping others. "Think of the things you can do, not what you can't do. If you focus on yourself, and think about the negative, it will make your condition worse. But if you focus on others, especially on how you can be an inspiration to them, then you've got to feel better, both physically and mentally."

In his introduction Michael spoke of "touching others' lives" and the importance of each one of us in effecting change in other people. Robert Frost's "The Road not Taken" shows us that when we touch so many other lives each fork in the road becomes one more chance to make a difference. Bebe Green touches us all with a message, not only of hope, but of inspiration, and not only inspiration from her to us, but how we can be an inspiration to others.

SQUARE ONE PRINCIPLES

Now that we've answered some important questions, and seen how at least one person applied these answers to her challenge of arthritis, let's examine some basic principles to consider in the application of your answers to the questions of *who, what, where, when,* and *why.*

Be Patient and Realistic

In assessing your new life, taking stock of what you've got to work with, and learning about your body all over again, one warning prevails: you have to think realistically and be patient. There were days when I felt really great and days when I felt really bad. It wasn't at all unusual for me to go for long periods without seeing any progress. I was always asking myself questions like: Will I ever get better? Will I see any progress today? You've got to keep the light at the end of the tunnel, but each step along the way has to be dealt with realistically. The only thing you can really do is start each day with the hope of being able to accomplish whatever it is you would like, and give it a try. But if it doesn't work out, then you take stock at the end of the day and try again the next. Having arthritis taught me how important patience is in the daily program. Dealing with getting well has to do with dealing with patience over the long haul.

Visualize Yourself as You Want to Be

When I look back on what happened to me there is one word that comes to mind—attitude. It's all attitude. I never gave up. I never lost sight of seeing myself again being well. I always pictured myself getting up and jogging again, or riding a bike to Mt. Wilson, or swimming again a pool. I visualized myself as I wanted to be. It doesn't just happen. You have to make it happen. You have to put all the pieces in the right place. You visualize yourself winning the race, or running again, or whatever it is you want to do, and keep that image in mind every day. You create a very idealistic situation for yourself. Put in as many positive thoughts as possible and keep out as many negative thoughts as possible.

Temper this with a dash of realism, of course. There will be many times when that mental attitude—that visualization—is nothing more than the daily routines of life: seeing yourself get out of bed, taking a shower, fixing breakfast, driving to work, doing your job, walking out to get the mail, going shopping, walking the dog, picking up the kids from school, cleaning house, and so on. What arthritis does is remind you of how many "little" things we all do every day of our lives that we used to take for granted—sort of like how you never realized how many times you swallow in a day until you get a sore throat. By visualizing those goals and keeping focused on them with a positive attitude, there is a greater chance of realizing them.

Become a Participant

The challenge of arthritis is to move from being a spectator to being a participant again. A spectator is one who might be told "there is no hope, go home and take these pills, follow instructions, and don't make waves." A participant is one who says, "I don't care what anyone says. No one knows my body as well as I do. Therefore I'm going to be the best I can be. I'm going to try. I'm not going to be afraid to give it my all." The key to this book, and the key to dealing with arthritis, is the mental challenge. The rest will follow. If the challenge were just a physical one, it would be easy—just take this drug, or whatever, and that's all. But that's not the way arthritis is—it requires work. You have to train your mind on how to deal with your body. And the key to training your mind is believing in yourself.

Be an M.V.P.

The first and perhaps most important step in developing a strong mental attitude to deal with arthritis is a sound and stable belief in yourself. Believing in yourself means feeling worthy of your dreams and goals. We all have the right to feel worthy of anything in life if you feel good about yourself. We all have the right to be an M.V.P., a *Most Valuable Person*. Many people feel they don't deserve the better things in life. But life is full of opportunity for everyone. That's why I deal with arthritis in an opportunistic way. I thought I was worthy of being better than this disease was letting me feel. I believed highly in myself and that I was worth the effort to do whatever it took to get better. It comes down to feeling that you yourself are worth the time and effort to get the best out of life.

Structure a Positive Environment

What about people who don't already feel positive about themselves? How do you learn to believe in yourself and feel worthy of your dreams and goals? The key is in structuring your environment so that you can't help but feel worthy. Surround yourself with people who are supportive. Get a job that you enjoy and makes you feel good. Ask your family to give you positive feedback. Teach them about arthritis so that they can understand what you are going through.

You should make a mental checklist for your environment. Try to make everything in your environment positive and attempt to eliminate all the negatives. We are not born with self-worth. It comes from the environment, so build your environment as positively as possible. Remind yourself of your goals and worthiness by surrounding yourself with successful people. This may even take the form of putting up posters and pictures of successful people and individuals who are high achievers. Seeing a picture of a successful individual, for instance, keeps you focused on the task at hand. What it says to me is, "If he did it, then so can I. He's a human being. I'm a human being. If he is successful, then there is no reason I can't be as well."

I have pictures of General George S. Patton. Michael has a poster of Einstein. Positive people serve as positive role models. Negative reminders make negative role models. It's not that you want to necessarily emulate these people. I don't want to be a general in the army. But you can identify with their strength and character, their energy and focus on their goals.

Why? Because they've been there. They know what it's like to be successful and you can know that too. These people have that karma, that aura about them, that says they are successful. Surround yourself with things that make you feel good, and you will feel good. Surround yourself with things that make you feel bad, and you will feel bad. When I got out of the hospital one of the first people I called was Michael, because ever since I've known him he's been a positive, uplifting person. When I went to him I knew he wouldn't say, "Oh George, you look terrible. There's no hope." If you talk to people who say things like that, you begin to believe it. The trick is to stack the deck on your side—the positive side. Life is a deck of cards—it might be aces or it might be jokers. Try to deal yourself into a royal flush. If it doesn't come out that way the first time, then reshuffle the deck until you get what you want.

Make Things Happen, Don't Let Them Happen to You

When I got arthritis I then began to realize just how many people don't feel good about themselves. I don't just mean arthritics, but everyone. They don't reach their potential because they don't believe in themselves. They don't feel they have the value to go to higher levels, be that emotional, physical, financial, or whatever. Some people put bumper stickers on their cars that say "_ _ _ _ happens." For these folks, that is usually what they get out of life. The "_ _ _ _ happens" philosophy tells these people that they can't control their lives, bad things will inevitably happen to them, and they can't do anything about it. This type of thinking destroys you mentally. You need to make things happen. Take action, not inaction. If you wait for things to happen to you, they will, and not necessarily in your favor. If you make things happen, they will, usually in your favor.

Give Yourself a Pat on the Back

Finally, take the time to appreciate the progress you have been making, and the steps you have accomplished. In other words, give yourself a pat on the back. Be kind to yourself. Work hard, but stop to appreciate the work you have done.

Take a moment at the end of the day to look back at what you did since that morning, and give yourself some positive strokes for a job well done. For most of us, the arthritis challenge means getting through the daily routines that so many take for granted. But don't just take it for granted. Take it for all it's worth. You've come back from square one and now you are ready to move ahead. So in the next chapter we will lay out a goal-setting program that will take you from here to there, wherever it is you want to go.

CHAPTER

7

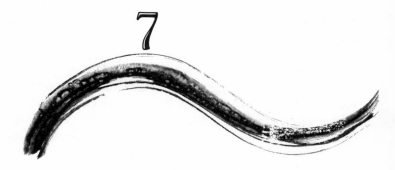

Your Arthritis Program: Setting Goals

"The greatest part of all the mischief in the world arises from the fact that men do not sufficiently understand their own aims. They have undertaken to build a tower, and spend no more labor on the foundation than would be necessary to erect a hut."

—JOHANN WOLFGANG VON GOETHE

Goethe's metaphor for success in life in general, and arthritic health in particular, is the core of this chapter, which in turn is the heart of this book: *laying the foundation* in order to build towers instead of huts. In order to achieve success in whatever you desire, you have to make that commitment to lay the foundation for your health and happiness and build that foundation as strong as you can. Once you've got that foundation, you can start designing your program for where you want to go in life.

This advice may seem simple enough. But it isn't unusual for simple ideas to be misunderstood or ignored. The key to not falling into the trap of missing the impact of simple ideas is found in Goethe's first sentence: *understanding your aims.* This may be translated into four simple ingredients: (1) writing down goals; (2) selecting different categories of goals; (3) ranking goals in a range from high to low; and (4) selecting a time frame in which to achieve these goals. Having a fix on your aims through setting goals will allow you to prepare a foundation for erecting towers, not huts.

*   *   *

For Martha Cooley—mother of four, department secretary for professors of history at Claremont Graduate School, and diagnosed with a progressive case of osteoarthritis—the key to dealing with this disease is understanding that "the bottom line is that you have to learn to live with arthritis by setting a sequence of goals from small to large, in order to structure a positive environment to learn to live with pain and fatigue." But Martha wants to pull no punches. Her unique way of dealing with arthritis—by being as mentally active as possible in order to distract her mind from the pain—does not eliminate the problem but optimizes the way she deals with it. "I think you can overcome a lot of pain by focusing on other things. You can override pain, assuming it is not too excruciating, by redirecting your mind toward something positive. For me, these things are primarily my goals, whether it is to take a trip to Hawaii or finish an afghan blanket."

As we shall see at the end of this chapter, the techniques Martha has developed for learning to live with arthritis follow the basic structure of your arthritis program: setting goals in order to lay a strong foundation. So we shall first examine the principles in general, followed by a closer look at Martha's goal structure and the characteristic way she has learned to face the mental challenge of arthritis.

WRITING DOWN GOALS

The first step in setting goals is to *write them down*. I mean literally getting out a piece of paper and jotting down what it is you want out of life. (If writing is painful or difficult because of inflammation, have someone else write them down for you. You could also record them on tape, but the idea of writing down your goals is so that you can *see* them.) Make a list of your goals, sort of like a shopping list for life. At first I wrote down lots of basic goals, such as: "Learn to walk without help." "Be able to get through the day on the job without pain." "Extend my range of motion by 10 percent." "Increase the strength of my muscles by 20 percent." Writing down the goal of accomplishing whatever task you have established for yourself restructures your thinking from "I wonder *if* I can accomplish it" to "I wonder *how* I will accomplish it." Most successful people actually make lists of goals they want to achieve. They write down their goals on a pad of paper they keep in their purse or briefcase, or taped to the office wall, so they are reminded of their plan every day.

The principle behind writing down goals is found in the simplicity of Goethe's advice—it helps you understand your aims. Setting goals by writing them down establishes the parameters within which your mind will allow your body to perform. In this sense then, the higher you set your goals (within reason—more on this later) the greater will be your success. The more you aim for, the more you will get. This principle is applicable to all aspects of life, whether it's winning a race, setting a world record, making money, getting high grades in school, or maintaining your health and strength. It's an axiom that is as basic as making a shopping list. If you write down all the items you need before you go to the store, you come out of the store with all those items, and then some. If you don't make the list, you will likely forget some items and fall short of your goal.

The very process of writing down your goals is a very cathartic, emotional, healing experience. It makes you feel like you are accomplishing something toward improving your life, because the first step—writing down goals—is as simple as taking out that pen and paper and doing it. It gets so discouraging sometimes—the pain and stiffness, not being able to move as swiftly as you would like—that sometimes I write down my goals just to make myself feel good because I can actually see them, which means I've taken a step in the right direction.

SELECTING CATEGORIES OF GOALS

The second step should be selecting a *category of goals:* health, athletic, financial, career, school, domestic, intellectual, and others. Naturally you are probably mostly concerned initially with the first one—health—but I found that by concentrating on other goals as well, not only did my life improve overall, but I found my mind distracted away from the discomforts of my arthritis.

RANKING GOALS

After you've established your categories of goals, the next step is to rank them from high to low. Memphis State University sports psychologist, Andy Meyers, in his work with Olympic athletes, expands this to include a range from "dream goals to daily goals." For Meyers, "the dream goals can be as ambitious as you like, then scaled down from there toward more realistic limits." We might also call these the stepping-stone goals. After you've established your long-range, dream goals, you set up the smaller steps along the way. I actually keep a log of how I feel each day and week, and how I'm doing on my list of stepping-stone goals toward those bigger goals. Examples of stepping-stone goals for recovering from and dealing with arthritis might include:

Get your mobility back.

Once you regain your mobility, work on strength and flexibility.

Learn to walk without crutches or without a walker.

Take daily walks outside, around the house, around the block, or up a hiking trail in the local mountains or park.

Increase the distance of your daily walk, perhaps first walking a mile, then two, and so forth, up to walking 45 minutes to an hour each day.

Develop a series of exercises ranging from easy to more strenuous.

Do these exercises every day, stretching and exercising in order to increase your range of motion and strength.

Increase your range of motion by 10 percent one week.

Increase your range of motion by 20 percent the next week, and so on.

Increase your strength by 10 percent at the gym over the course of the first month.

Increase your strength by 20 percent over the course of the next few months, and so on.

The progression may take awhile, but when you have the smaller goals along the journey, it helps keep you focused on the immediate task, which would be more difficult if you only had that dream goal out there.

That's why it is really important to keep a chart of progress. You might actually use graph paper and mark how far your range of motion was for the day, or how far you walked, or how many laps you swam in the pool, or whatever it is you did. Then if you get hurt, or you don't feel too well, you can look back on the chart and see where you went wrong. Maybe you pushed yourself too much that week. The personal progress chart is your own unique system, designed specifically for you. There are no real guidelines in books on how much exercise you should do as an arthritic. You have to begin very gently and slowly, working with a therapist, and build up step by step to where you feel able to move on.

When I first got on a stationary bike at the rehabilitation center, for example, the chart said I should begin by riding 20 minutes. I didn't think I could make even 10 minutes, so I just got on and did the best I could do. I noted the time and mileage on my chart, and tried to do a little better the next day. There is a lot of trial-and-error experimenting. But the encouraging thing is that progress will come. If you stick to it you will see yourself getting better and better. I can guarantee that nothing feels better than seeing yourself making progress.

Ranking goals gets back to the "laying the foundation" principle. From your foundation, you have to then begin building the structure you want. But this doesn't come out of thin air by magically waving the wand. From your long-range goal you then need to be specific. Whether you want to rehabilitate yourself from arthritis to be able to run a marathon or run to your car, you don't just jump out of bed and run down the hall. First you have to get your health back. Then comes your flexibility. Then strength. You relearn to walk, then jog, then run. The immediate goals come first, then the long-range/dream goals. Dream goals are very personal. You affirm them to yourself. You have to have dreams. If we didn't have dreams we would live in a very dull, predictable world. We have to want to strive for things that seem to be out of reach. That's where we push ourselves to be better. Anything can happen. You never know. But if you don't dream it, it won't happen.

SELECTING A TIME FRAME

Along with ranking your goals from high to low, you also need to rank them by the time frame in which to achieve them. In general, the more basic goals are the daily goals, and the dream goals are the long-range goals. So we might design a time frame from daily goals, to weekly goals, to monthly goals, to yearly goals, to your long-range/dream goals. If you were writing these down, you might even have a separate page for each time frame—for example, a page of daily goals (which will change daily), and a page of weekly goals (which will change weekly). By writing this down you can chart your progress by seeing if those daily goals meet the weekly goals, and if the weekly goals meet the monthly goals, and so on.

Daily Goals

Each morning get up and check your list to see what is going to be done. This list should also include all the mundane things of life that have to be taken care of in order to accomplish your goal without losing your house, job, or spouse. A lot of people forget that before you go out to change the world you first have to take out the trash, do the dishes, clean the house, wash the car, and mow the lawn! These daily, routine goals of life everyone has to do in order to move upward to the weekly goals.

Weekly Goals

The weekly goals can be easily planned out on a piece of notebook paper every Sunday night. Just look at the calendar to see what is coming up, and make a list of items to be checked off as you accomplish each one. If you plan to ride the stationary bike at the gym for a certain length of time at a given level of difficulty, then you need to figure out how the time and levels will break down by the day.

Or perhaps you have a monthly goal of cleaning out and reorganizing the garage. Because of your arthritis, it might be a slow procedure. That means each week you should have some of it done. Set out a certain amount for each week so that by the end of the month it is finished. Of course, to complete the weekly task requires a daily goal list.

Monthly Goals

At the beginning of each month you should look at the calendar to see if one of your yearly goals falls within that period of time. If so, plan the month around that event. Build up your preparations with a plan to hit your peak on the day of that goal, whatever it is. If you were going to do a run or a bike ride, for example, decide how many miles you plan to ride for the entire month, so that the weekly goals can then be composed. For example, if you want to ride your bike 200 miles total in the month, then you will need to ride 50 miles each week.

Or perhaps you want to try to gain a certain range of motion in your arms by the end of the year. That means you should have a plan to reach a certain level by each month. When you look at your monthly goal list, you'll see how far you need to get that month and plan on reaching that level.

Yearly Goals

Yearly goals should be established on New Year's Day. The old "New Year's day resolution" is an excellent time to write down the goals for the year that will ultimately help you attain those long-range/dream goals. Decide what major events or things you want to accomplish for the upcoming year and mark them on the calendar. For example, maybe you want to take a trip to Europe or Hawaii in the summer. You will start building in January by setting this as your yearly goal. In order to meet this goal you will have to have monthly goals of saving a certain amount of money, purchasing the tickets by a specific date, making hotel reservations by another date, and so on.

Whatever it is you choose, make sure it is reasonably harder than what you are expecting to be able to accomplish, or what you've been told is your limitation. Remember, the purpose of setting goals is to reach out further than before. If it becomes too difficult or painful, you can always rewrite the goals more modestly. These lists are for your eyes only so there is nothing that says you can't change your mind. Also, don't choose too many goals for this list, or you may lose focus on the importance of each one.

Long-Range Goals

Long-range goals can and should include the ultimate levels of success which your wildest imaginations can conjure. This would be Meyers's "dream goal" concept. These might encompass anything you've always dreamed of doing, but never dared to hope could come true. Let these long-range goals be as wild and farfetched as you like. No one except you has to see this list. And remember, this list is a relative one. A basic goal for someone might be a dream goal for another. Examples might include staying fit for life, losing a certain amount of weight, building up your muscles and strength, and traveling to foreign lands. The most successful people I know all had dream goals long before they had any hint of being successful. Once again, the famous people we all admire were once unknowns, with dream goals that probably seemed unrealizable. But they made it and so can you!

*   *   *

These goal-setting principles in laying the foundation are pretty basic, yet you can't skip over them. Lying there in bed in the hospital I had to re-establish the ranking of my goals. You know what my dream goal was, but my immediate goal was trying to figure out how to get out of the bed. Nothing happens without that first step. I had to devise ways to keep from falling over when I was relearning to walk. Taking a shower had a whole new meaning. Driving a car, shopping, work—all had to be restructured in a goal pattern from small to large, and from immediate to long range.

Everything happens in a stepping-stone pattern: I've got to get out of bed. I've got to get to therapy. I've got to get mobility. I've got to get strength. With strength I can move better. Then I can get outside. Then I can start walking again. Then I can get my weight back. To reiterate, it's A to Z, and Z is the dream goal. But you don't just leap from A to Z, you have to go from A to B to C to D . . . and eventually you'll get there. It's work. You can't skip steps.

HAVING BASIC GOALS

Most arthritics, I realize, probably don't have some of the crazy goals I've had, as we'll see shortly in Martha Cooley's story. And that's O.K. The point is to have *some* goal that involves either physical exercise in order to keep your joints loose and your muscles and ligaments strong enough to support your body with minimal pain, or mental exercise to keep your mind off the arthritis and on something else.

Probably the biggest goal of most of the arthritics I know is to avoid feeling that constant, nagging pain. But the problem is they sit and think about it. Sometimes the best way to avoid the pain is to get up and *do* something about it. That pain drives them up the wall. It drove me up the wall, too. I know what it's like. But I stopped thinking about it. I made my pain part of my goal to feel better, because I knew that the pain of exercising would help attenuate the overall pain. And it did. So I mentally turned that whole physical scenario around. I knew I had to go through pain induced by myself, in order to alleviate the pain induced by the disease. Most arthritics are in a quagmire. They want to feel better but they haven't a clue on what to do about it. The mental challenge of arthritis is to clarify and execute a plan to deal with the disease.

BEING REALISTIC

One caveat should be noted here. The goals you set must be within reason. Establishing totally unrealistic goals may likely lead to total frustration. For 99 percent of the thousands of people who enter the New York Marathon, for example, it would be unrealistic to set a goal of winning the race. It would not be unrealistic, however, to set a goal of improving one's personal best by, say, 10 percent. Likewise, perhaps you want to learn to live a normal life without pain. It may be that this is impossible. A more realistic goal might be to *minimize* your pain, or *optimize* your movements. We all have built-in limitations and certain biological constraints which must be taken into consideration. But it is also true that very few of us have ever reached those limitations. Henry Ford once noted that "there isn't a man living who isn't capable of doing more than he thinks he can do." Establishing your goals can help you realize your limitations, which are likely to be much higher than you ever imagined.

THE VALUE OF SETTING GOALS

What we are doing here is striving for that goal of how to have more out of life and how to get to that point. That hinges on believing in yourself, of establishing that inner confidence we discussed in the previous chapter. Once you've got the rules of the mental challenge down then you will be more open to change and want to try things that lead to greater success.

This first step—laying the foundation through setting goals—is probably the most important in getting started in your new life. Your goal program is the superstructure of the rest of the mental challenge of catapulting yourself into higher levels of achievement and restoring your life. The rest of this book consists of subdivisions of this larger super-structure that will become the guideline of your life. Always come back to your chart—your mental game plan—to rein-force your actions, to make modifications as necessary, and to keep a focus on *why* your actions are directed as they are, and *how* it is you will accomplish what you have set out for yourself.

CREATIVE STRUCTURING: HOW MARTHA COOLEY DEALS WITH ARTHRITIS

Sometime around 1970, when she was in the early stages of raising a family and developing a career, Martha Cooley be-gan to get a little pain in her feet. In time, the little pain spread into her ankles, knees, and eventually even up to her hips. She finally found a doctor who gave her an explanation that made some sense, but left her with little to do about it: she was told she had "a little arthritis." I don't know if hav-ing "a little arthritis" is like being "a little pregnant," but one similarity is certain: either you are or you are not. And if you are, you know it almost immediately.

By 1988 Martha's arthritis had spread to her upper body, attacking the joints in her shoulders, arms, wrists, and fin-gers. The diagnosis grew in intensity along with the disease, from "a little arthritis" to "osteoarthritis." For the past two years she has experienced a significant increase in pain and inflammation, accompanied by a reduction in physical move-ment and activity. This has required a corresponding change in techniques of how to deal with the severity of the disease. But for an optimist like Martha Cooley, an increase in pain just means an increase in mental toughness. "My motto is never, never, never, never give up. Each day I structure my activities to motivate myself. You've got to pull yourself up by the bootstraps and try again and again, each day.

For Martha this means setting goals to structure her environment, both physically and mentally, to optimize her arthritis challenge in her favor. For example, when she gets dressed in the morning she lays out all her clothes and shoes in one place, then puts everything on at one time, rather than sitting down, getting up to go to the other closet, then sitting down again, getting up again, and so forth. "The point is to structure the environment for efficiency. I try to get the most number of things done in the shortest amount of time and with the least amount of movement. For example, I've rearranged my kitchen for maximum efficiency by putting the most-used dishes within easy reach, heavier pots and pans down below so I don't have to reach up to lift a heavy object, lighter objects like cups and glasses higher up, and so forth.

At work, where she manages an office full of history professors at Claremont Graduate School, Martha maximizes her time and minimizes her movements in her program of efficiency. Working on the second story of a two-story building, Martha plans her day so that she doesn't have to make numerous trips up and down the stairs. "I organize things so that when I do go downstairs to photocopy something, I'll wait until I have other things to do, like going by the administration office or the mail room. With osteoarthritis, the pain and inflammation is very fatiguing, and since having an active career is important to me, I must plan my work so I can last the whole day and not tire out."

As Martha's osteoarthritis worsened, even driving long distances became a problem. "If I drove for any length of time at all it became very difficult to 'unlock' my body in trying to get out of the car." Therefore, Martha and her family moved to a location closer to her work so that she now only has to drive five miles each way. "Again, the point is conservation of energy. Minimize stress and maximize relaxation."

Like anyone else, of course, Martha has her days when the efficiency program falls apart, or the arthritis symptoms flare up unbearably, and she gets discouraged. "Oh sure, I get depressed like anyone else. It comes from realizing you have a disease that can be treated but never cured. There are days when you realize you've got this thing for life, and if you think about it too long, it can get really depressing." How does she overcome this depression? "I try not to dwell on it. I focus on other things. The last supervisor I had taught me to *focus, focus, focus.*"

Martha focuses on expressing herself creatively through artistic projects like needlecraft and crocheting. She weaves afghan blankets of various colors and designs. "This expression takes your mind off the pain. Having the goal of completing some creative project keeps me focused on the goal rather than the pain. If I didn't do this I'd drive both myself and my family crazy."

The key to Martha's success, therefore, lies in what we've been discussing in this chapter: laying the foundation through setting goals. "I have have a whole bunch of small, short-term goals that I use to keep myself occupied and not thinking about my arthritis. Some of them are kind of silly, but they work. For instance, I've got this cat that I've worked to teach lots of tricks. They say you can't teach cats tricks, so I made it my goal to teach my cat some tricks. Now this cat rolls over and even falls down and plays dead when I point my finger at it and say 'bang'! To be honest, it's pretty hard to feel bad when your cat is so playful. Pets just lift you up because they are always so happy."

On the other end of the goal spectrum, Martha has her dream and long-range goals. One goal she has had for a while is to travel to Hawaii, so she is saving her money and making plans to try to make it to the islands sometime next year. "The very process of visualizing myself in Hawaii, relaxing on a beach and enjoying the warm weather, makes my bones feel better! Another long-range goal she recently established is poetry. "I saw an advertisement for a poetry contest, so I decided I would give it a shot. Why not? I wrote one and took it to the poet laureate on campus at one of the Claremont colleges. He told me it needed improvement, but had great promise. For me, this was a great victory, I hadn't expected anything."

Herein lies a perfect example of how the mind works on the body. Upon this professor's pronouncement of praise on Martha's poetry, she immediately felt physically better. "I came home and vacuumed, cleaned the house, got things organized. I had so much energy that day! Positive feedback from people make you feel physically stronger." The point is to seek out and find ways to make yourself feel better. This is what Martha means by structuring your environment and setting goals in a positive direction. "Life does not come knocking on your door to hand you what you need. It is an active process of setting goals that will make your life positive. When things get tense at the office or at home, I listen to music, read, do needlework—relaxing sorts of things. I structure my environment to be as uplifting and rewarding as possible."

Martha makes another interesting observation about being active that I hadn't thought of before. She says that activity and mobility is as much a mental process as it is a physical one. "Mobility is a state of mind. Even if you are in a wheelchair you can be mobile—you might be mentally mobile, but it is still mobility. What I mean is staying mentally focused on positive, active sorts of things. For example, the reason I like working at a college is because of the students. They are young and so full of energy and spirit, excitement and new ideas. They are flexible and challenging. And all of this makes me feel young, energetic, excited, and challenged."

Martha offers other suggestions for small goals and ways to structure your environment to make life easier. "When the pain is continuous you have to break it up or you will go nuts. Pick up the phone and call a friend you haven't talked to for some time. That will take your mind off the pain. Or take a nice hot shower. Or fix yourself a delicious meal. Anything to break the cycle of pain. Again, the bottom line is to face the fact that you've got arthritis; there is no cure, so learn to live with it by fixing things to optimize your life."

The importance of Martha's message is *not* that goal setting and positive environmental structuring will relieve your arthritis pain. The point is that such *mental* activities will redirect your attention away from the *physical* distraction of pain. Arthritis is initially a physical challenge, but it isn't long before it becomes a mental challenge. The key lies in turning the mental challenge into one that you can manage, rather than one that manages you. It is a matter of control, and Martha serves as a fine example of someone who has taken control of her arthritis.

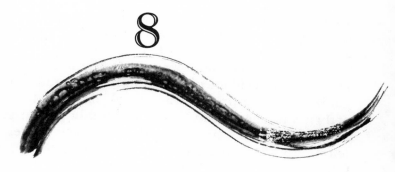

Your Arthritis Program: Attaining Your Goals

"If to do were as easy as to know what were good to do, chapels had been churches, and poor men's cottages princes' palaces."

—SHAKESPEARE, *THE MERCHANT OF VENICE*

Now that you've established your goals, you've committed yourself to meeting the challenge: *attaining those goals.*

The problem with having arthritis, of course, is that it puts you in a totally new environment, with a new set of circumstances that you have to deal with accordingly. While attaining goals might have been easy before, now even easy goals can be difficult to achieve. When you get arthritis, you have to create new standards because you are dealt a whole new set of circumstances. Therefore, while it may be easy to write down your new goals, attaining them will be an unaccustomed experience for you, requiring an unfamiliar set of standards of what it means to be successful.

Take Amye Leong, for example, the founder of Young at Heart and president of the American Juvenile Arthritis Organization. Before she was struck down with rheumatoid arthritis at age 19, Amye was incredibly active: golf, tennis, swimming, high school homecoming queen, college debating team, student president of her dorm at the University of California, Santa Barbara. You name it, she did it, and with gusto. Rheumatoid arthritis brought her activities, energies, and spirit to a screeching halt. She dropped from 110 pounds to 79 pounds. Her joints swelled beyond belief. When she could still walk, she was hunched over, barely able to scoot her feet along the ground. But soon enough she couldn't even do that. Wheelchair-bound, and finally bedridden, Amye couldn't perform the simplest of tasks, such as feeding herself. She went two years without even being able to comb the back of her hair.

But then Amy began a long and painful comeback that eventually got her on crutches, and finally to where she could walk again unaided. Gone were the days of free-swinging activities and endless energy, but Amye designed new goals, and developed completely new methods of attaining those goals. It was no longer just a matter of setting her sights on what she wanted and going out to get it. Now she plans carefully, paces her energy, plots her days to be as goal-oriented as she ever was before, but in a whole new way. Amye is as active as she ever was, but as she has discovered, being active is also a state of mind.

In this chapter I will review the principles of your arthritis program: attaining your goals, and then return to the incredible story of Amye Leong, and how she has structured her environment to be able to attain all her goals in spite of one of the severest cases of rheumatoid arthritis I've ever seen.

A NEW DEFINITION OF WINNING

When I grew up Vince Lombardi, the coach of the Green Bay Packers football team, had a saying that became famous throughout the sporting world: "Winning isn't everything, it's the only thing." I believe this is only partially correct. Winning is the only thing, but it depends on how you define winning. The criteria for judging can come from two sources: others and yourself.

We usually think of winning as being first. But that leaves out everyone else in the competition. A new definition of winning might be: To win is to perform at the highest level you are capable of reaching, to use every resource available to you, and to give 100 percent of your energy and effort to the task at hand. If it happens that someone else has also done this, and his or her capabilities are higher than yours, then there is only one conclusion: you both won. Your opponent just happened to cross the line ahead of you. Your respect for that person, and for yourself, should be elevated.

The underlying premise is trying your best. Don't ever leave yourself being a "wanna be," or a "wish I could'a been" person. Winning means having no regrets—knowing that you gave it everything you had. This principle of success is especially important for individuals with arthritis. Since no one but yourself really knows what you are going through, and how arthritis has affected you specifically, only you can be the judge of how successful you were in attaining your goals. To allow others to be your *sole* guideline of how you judge your own success can be very defeating. To use outside sources as the touchstone of achievement is to put your own self-esteem in others' hands.

RUNNING THE RACE
AGAINST YOURSELF

It is true that we establish our parameters of success through the experience of interacting with others. But the more important (and difficult) understanding of your capacities comes from pushing yourself higher and higher against *your own* established limits. Comparing your results only with others, rather than your own abilities, can lead to much frustration. You must figure out what your typical level of performance is, especially now that you have re-assessed your new physical parameters, and compare results with this mark, not your greatest performance or the best results of others.

When I got out of the hospital and started learning to get around again, I expected to be able to do things as well as I did them before. I think everyone does this, because there is a certain amount of denial going on. You just don't want to believe you have a lifelong crippling disease. You expect to recover, as you would from most illnesses and diseases, and return to normal. With arthritis it just isn't that way. You have to keep in mind that you will have ups and downs throughout the year, and performance in whatever you are doing must be compared to the normal day, not the exceptional.

Regardless of the severity of the task—easy or hard—if you've done your best you should be satisfied with the results, absolute or relative. It may be that just cooking a meal or driving a car is now an acomplishment. If so, then relish the success of such tasks as they are done. You can work up to bigger and better things later on—those long-range and dream goals. In the meantime, be your own judge and standard. What it comes down to is that you have to answer to yourself. The bottom line is your gut feeling and what your heart tells you—how *you* feel, not anyone else. You run the race of life against yourself. As Benjamin Franklin noted in *Poor Richard's Almanack:* "Strive to be the greatest man in your country, and you may be disappointed; Strive to be the best and you may succeed. He may well win the race that runs by himself."

A MONOMANIAC WITH A MISSION

In order to achieve your goals it helps to be really interested in them. You have to want to do them. Nobody can tell you which goals you want. A chart can't tell you to do them. You have to have that inner drive, that willpower, to be able to want to follow through. Inner drive is related to interest in achieving your goals and the belief that these goals will be positive for you, that they will benefit you, and that they won't be a waste of time. If you know your goals will improve your life, you will be more motivated to accomplish them. If you think that your goal will help you attenuate your arthritis symptoms, or help you deal with your arthritis in trying to live a normal life, then you will be much more interested in pursuing that goal. I knew that exercise and stretching would improve the range of motion of my arms and legs, and that this in turn would make it easier for me to walk, drive, and just get around at the house or on the job. So even though exercising and stretching really hurt sometimes, I pushed myself anyway because I knew it was good for me.

In this pursuit of your goals there is one word that best describes the person who is most likely to attain his aspirations. According to Jay Snelson that word is *monomaniacal.* Mono means "one." Maniacal meas "ungovernable excitement." The *Oxford English Dictionary* defines *monomaniacal* as "an exaggerated enthusiasm for or devotion to one subject." In the quest for your objectives you should be monomaniacal. Sometimes I call it monofanatical. The principle is the same: pursue your goal with a relentless energy that can carry you through the many obstacles, physical and psychological, that will arise. The greater your enthusiasm, the more powerful will be your ability to leap over these hurdles. The inflamed joints, the injuries, the general pain, cold weather, and the boredom of the daily routine that everyone experiences, will be easier to deal with when maintaining a high level of enthusiasm. The famed management consultant and entrepreneurial professor from Claremont Graduate School, Peter Drucker, noted that "whenever anything is being accomplished, it is being done, I have learned, by a monomaniac with a mission."

Be Passionate for Life

So the basic premise here is that it will be much easier to accomplish your goals if you are monomaniacal. But how does one become monomaniacal? Can you get a monomaniacal pill at the store? Can you get a monomaniacal injection at the doctors? Of course not. You don't become monomaniacal, since such personality traits probably cannot be learned. You find something you are already passionate about. Discover that one thing you love to do more than anything else—your life's dream—and a monomaniacal pursuit of that quest will come naturally.

One of the hallmarks of successful individuals, in any field, is that they are passionate in their pursuit of excellence. They love what they are doing and would do it even if it weren't their profession. It's what we might call the lottery test: If you won the lottery how would your life change? If you answer that you would quit everything you are doing and change your whole life, you probably aren't doing what you really want to do. If you answer that you would continue doing what you are doing (with some slight modifications such as an increased standard of living), you probably are doing that which is your own best destiny. The key is finding a way to do what you love to do in the most likely case scenario that you don't win the lottery. If you can manage that then pursuing your goals with a monomaniacal passion will come easily and naturally. You don't have to *learn* to be monomaniacal—you will be.

When you have a passion in what you believe, that passion is what keeps you consistent. You like who you are and what you are doing so you want to continue doing what you are doing. In this sense, then, life is a continuation of passion—a passion for your mate, a passion for your family, a passion for your job. You have to really want to be involved. A participant is passionate. A spectator is passive.

Reading of the passion someone has for his career, the zest an individual feels for his life's work, the fervor a person holds for his one unerring vision of the world, or the ecstasy one feels when he catches his dream stirs a deep energy inside our souls. Read the following passage, for example, from Duke Ellington's autobiography, *Music is My Mistress:*

> I live a life of primitivity with the mind of a child and an unquenchable thirst for sharps and flats. . . . Living in a cave, I am almost a hermit, but there is a difference, for I have a mistress. Lovers have come and gone, but only my mistress stays. She is beautiful and gentle. She waits on me hand and foot. She is a swinger. She has grace. To hear her speak, you can't believe your ears. She is ten thousand years old. She is as modern as tomorrow, a brand-new woman every day, and as endless as time mathematics. Living with her is a labyrinth of ramifications. I look forward to her every gesture. Music is my mistress, and she plays second fiddle to no one.

If you have a passion like this it will keep you strong, and other people will pick up on that and want to be around you. It's contagious. Life is a puzzle and you have to put the pieces in place. But you have to want it to be the best damn puzzle you ever made for yourself.

Be Passionate but Not Obsessive

Yet you have to strike a balance in what you are doing so you are not obsessive or compulsive. The passion gives you direction, and balance enables you to do it enough to be successful, yet not so much that you neglect other important areas in your life. You certainly don't want to become so obsessed with a goal that you sacrifice family, spouse, or job.

The line between passion and obsession is having a balance of passions. You can have a lot of passions, not just one. I like talking to my customers—that's a passion. It's my job, but it's also my passion. That's what keeps me going out day after day. Financial security it a passion of mine, so that my family doesn't have to worry. I have a passion for my fiancée, my dog, my hobbies, my sports. I have a passion for my friends. Passion is also a belief in yourself. Your attitude is a passion. Multiple passions are healthy.

What can be dangerous is monopassions. For example, just focusing on making money but neglecting other, important passions can be unhealthy. And with this balance, failing in one is not nearly so bad when you have other passions to fall back on.

Create an Environment for Passion

The frustrations that arthritis can cause, of course, can make being passionate for your goals difficult. Therefore you need all the help you can get. What I suggest is creating an environment that you really like, that sets you up to have a passion for your goals. Your job, your family, your mate, your car, your house, everything—if you really like what you're doing, the goal achievement comes easier. It helps to surround yourself with people who are supportive, with friends and family members who, though they may not have arthritis, understand the pain you are going through. To the extent that we are all very much a product of our environments, why not set up yours to be as positive and uplifting as possible?

Regardless of what you do, however, passion can wane in due course, and it will be easier to maintain your focus if you remember that all goals will take time and energy to reach, and the higher the goal, the more effort required. The earlier in the game you are, the more energy you will have to invest in order to see results later down the line. The curve below describes this phenomenon. John Marino, the founder of the Race Across America, uses this curve to demonstrate the principle that success does not come overnight.

THE GOAL ATTAINMENT CURVE

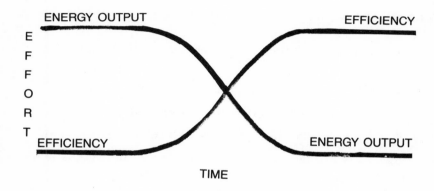

At the beginning of any endeavor a tremendous amount of energy must be invested to get started. Likewise, the results will be relatively paltry. In business, for example, it takes years of working long days to start your own company and see it succeed. But eventually the amount of energy investment will decrease and efficiency will rise. If you are struggling to deal with arthritis and your goal is to improve a significant amount—say, in your ability to move around reasonably well without too much pain—in the beginning you will have to expend tremendous amounts of energy because your body is not efficient. As you get in better shape, gain muscle weight, increase cardiovascular capacity, and improve the range of motion of your arms and legs, your body becomes more efficient and energy expenditure decreases.

The importance of this goal attainment curve is to keep in mind that early in your quest you may not see the amount of progress you would like see. But by maintaining a passionate and monomaniacal drive toward your goal, in time the energy curve will decrease while the efficiency curve will increase. Don't quit before you have reached the level where the curves cross and success becomes imminent. Persistence is everything.

TEN REASONS WHY PEOPLE ATTAIN THEIR GOALS:

1. They write their goals down so they don't forget them.

2. They focus on their goals every day.

3. They select goals that they enjoy pursuing.

4. They pursue their goals with a relentless passion.

5. They are flexible enough to change their goals when necessary.

6. They do not let a failure slow them down.

7. They learn from failures.

8. They maintain a sense of balance between work, play, and relaxation.

9. They keep a sense of humor and playfulness in whatever they are doing.

10. They are always growing, learning, and bettering themselves.

TEN REASONS WHY PEOPLE DO NOT ATTAIN THEIR GOAL

1. They have no goals, or don't write them down.

2. Therefore they have nothing to focus on, and therefore become distracted.

3. They treat their work or job as drudgery instead of joy.

4. They are not excited about their goals.

5. They lack creative imagination in developing solutions to problems.

6. They are crushed when they fail.

7. They do not learn from failures.

8. They let the environment control them, instead of vice versa.

9. They lack joy, happiness, and a sense of fun in their lives.

10. They give up when the going gets tough.

KNOWING YOUR LIMITATIONS: AMYE LEONG ON ATTAINING GOALS

All principles need examples, and I can't think of a better one than Amye Leong, an individual who has redefined the concept of goal attainment better than anyone I know. Because of the severity of her arthritis, Amye has had to constantly redefine her goals, reassess her abilities and limitations, and generally learn to set daily goals with long-range goals in mind, but always remembering that because her arthritis is so variable her goals must be also.

Since the age of 19, when she was officially diagnosed as having rheumatoid arthritis (she is currently 34), Amye has experienced *nine* joint replacement operations, a situation so difficult to face that she often uses humor to deal with it ("2bionic" reads her automobile license plate!). "My arthritis began in my chest, specifically in my sternum, when I was 17 years old. My doctor told me it was overwork and stress, and so gave me a shot of cortisone, but within a few days the pain came back and was so bad that it brought tears to my eyes just to breathe."

It wasn't long before the pain spread to her arms and legs, but like many young people who get arthritis, it was a year and a half before Amye was properly diagnosed. The associations with old age makes arthritis in the young difficult to diagnose. Often the patient herself doesn't realize it, or even denies the possibility. "Denial is a bigger problem in young populations than old because they don't expect to get arthritis. Arthritis is supposed to be an old person's disease."

Because of this, in 1984 Amye founded Young at Heart, an organization to help young people with arthritis communicate with each other and network across the United States. The organization has now blossomed into a group with over 500 members in Southern California alone. "When I founded this group I couldn't even walk. I was still in a wheelchair. People looked at me like a cripple and treated me like a cripple. I began to believe it myself. But when I discovered there were others like me, I realized how helpful it was just to know that. It is very cathartic to share with others the facts and pains of this disease."

Amye's influence has spread. As far as she knows there are at least eight or nine other groups in the United States that have developed since she founded her group. Plus, she now travels to Washington, D.C. every year to attend conferences and meetings of the National Council on Self-help and Public Health, of which she serves as chairman, advising the Surgeon General on how best to incorporate self-help groups into our national health system. "When you go to the doctor he sees you for 15 minutes. You can't expect him to solve all your problems in that amount of time. Self-help groups, like Young at Heart, are critical for getting people back on their feet. Young at Heart is particularly important in meeting the needs of a very particular group—the young. Most arthritis self-help groups feature people over 60 years old. The subjects they are interested in and the problems they address are just not appropriate for a 19-year-old kid."

OVERCOMING SPECIAL PROBLEMS
OF ARTHRITIS

Herein lies the message that Amye brings to the subject of goal attainment—determining exactly what problems you want to address, what goals you want to set, and then finding out what others have done to meet these goals. "Before I got arthritis I was totally goal-oriented and very passionate about everything I did. Arthritis took this away from me, and I've had to fight to get it back. I had to be excited about life to find my purpose again. It was like my life ended and I had to start over. Knowing that others went through the same thing helped me realize I could do it. I think this is what is behind the national movement of self-help groups in all fields. It means discovering you are not alone, and then finding out what others do to solve the same problems you've got. People that share similar problems gain strength from networking and communicating."

Amye is swift to point out that this networking does not require some altruistic giving of yourself. In fact, she says, "what you discover is that by helping others you are really helping yourself. It feels good to tell someone how you deal with arthritis. It helps them and it helps you." What sorts of problems does Amye address in her group meetings? The widest variety imaginable, for example:

DATING. "The anxiety over dating is tremendous. The cause of this is low self-esteem. Arthritis can make you feel less confident, which makes it difficult to feel good about going out with other people. What I advise is honesty. Don't try to hide your arthritis from someone you are going out with, because they will pick up cues and infer other things. When they don't realize someone has arthritis, many people think that the person is just lazy because he moves slowly. Then they think negative things, because being lazy is looked down upon in our culture. But when most people find out you've got arthritis, they are much more sympathetic."

In fact, Amye recalls the night she met her fiancé. Her girlfriend had been trying to talk her into getting out for quite some time, but Amye didn't want to go because she didn't feel good about herself. Finally, reluctantly, she agreed to go to a party on the condition that her girlfriend help her walk in and sit down so that she wouldn't have to use her crutches. Then no one would know she had a problem. They went to the party, and Amye managed to get to a sitting position, where she remained. A gentleman talked with her for a long time, until the party was over and it was time to leave. Amye tried to walk out with him to her car, but it became obvious to him that something was wrong. "I had been sitting for so long that I was 'locked up' and could hardly move without extreme pain. But I didn't want to say anything, so I gritted my teeth and started to get up. I was moving really slow. I began to sweat because I was working so hard. Finally he asked if I was okay, so I told him I had 'a touch of arthritis.' He said he knew about that because he worked with horses and when they got 'a touch of arthritis' they could hardly move. So he knew the problem was more serious than that, and practically carried me out to the car. He was sensitive and understanding, and this is why I think honesty is the best way to deal with the problem."

SEX.   Hardly anyone talks about sex and arthritis, but it is a real problem that Amye deals with in her workshops at Young at Heart, and more than a passing number of kids are interested in it. "Let's face it. Humans are sexual beings, and I don't care what age you are, you're never too old for sex." Even though Amye's group ranges in age from 16 to 40, she is quick to note that the sex and arthritis question is certainly not limited to this group. "Basically, without getting too graphic, I tell them where there is a will there is a way. If you and your partner desire a sexual relationship, you will find a way to make it happen. Attitude and determination are the keys to recovery and rehabilitation in all aspects of arthritis, and the same applies here." Amye also notes that the sex question is not limited to the physical. Sexuality is also a state of mind that deals with attraction, attitude, as well as technique and position. "Our goal is to first build self-esteem. Once you've got your confidence back, the sexuality will come naturally."

ACTIVITIES AND EXERCISE.   For many arthritics, the disease means a significant curtailment of pre-arthritis activity levels. There are, after all, certain physical limitations that may not be overcome no matter how hard you want it. But Amye notes that activities and exercise are not just physical but mental as well. "Being active is a state of mind. You can be every bit the participant you ever were, just on a different level. For example, I can't play volleyball anymore because I can't swing my arm over my head, but I can sure as heck go to the game, keep score, root and cheer, laugh and have fun, and go out with everyone after the game. I call that being active." She extends athletics to the mind. "You can be an intellectual athlete. Use your brain. Do things that require thinking. Arthritis can't get into your brain!"

FAMILIES.   Another problem Amye addresses is how families should deal with children and adolescents who have arthritis, or how the kids should deal with their parents who get arthritis. "How should a parent encourage little Johnny to be all he can be when what he thinks is important is being physically able to participate on the playground with the other boys? I suggest that the parents encourage their children to develop interests in areas that are not so physically demanding, like indoor games, or computers. I'm telling you, the computer has been the greatest boon for children's intellect ever. It can hold their attention for hours, and they have to use their brain to the fullest. Computers are a great substitute for the playground. You don't have to climb the jungle gym to be a worthwhile child."

DEPRESSION.   One of the biggest problems Amye encounters with arthritics of all ages is depression. The causes can be varied and complex, but the root cause is usually the same: "The realization that you have a crippling disease that probably won't go away can surely get you down. For me, the most depressing aspect of arthritis is the fatigue factor. Arthritis can be very tiring so that even the most humdrum daily chores are magnified beyond all proportions. Sometimes I have to take naps in the afternoon to get through the day. If I have to sit in meetings all day, every day for a week, like when I go to Washington, D.C., it takes me days to recover when I return."

Amye also notes that depressions can get extremely serious. "We've had several cases of depression so serious that suicide seemed an option to a couple of these kids. Depression can sometimes also lead to drug addiction because that becomes an easy out for dealing with the pain. In reality, of course, this only makes it worse. This is why I use humor therapy. You've got to look at life with a certain amount of playfulness and fun, or your arthritis can really get you down. Funny movies and books, records and tapes, comedy clubs, and just plain laughing with your friends can sure make you feel better."

GOAL ATTAINMENT.   "Arthritis has changed my goals. I've always been a goal-directed person; I've just redirected them from the physical to the intellectual. The key to getting your goals is knowing your limitations, and knowing when to stop and when to go again. Goal setting is one thing, but you will fail if you don't know your limitations. I wish there were a little bell in my brain that went off to tell me that I had one hour left before I tire out so that I could paced myself. Unfortunately there is no such bell, and because arthritis is such a variable disease, it is sometimes hard to know when to say 'when.' So I set my goals with reasonable expectations, and am always willing and able to change them if necessary. For example, if I am going out for a while with friends, I make sure they know that I might have to go home early, just in case. Or, take a simple goal like going shopping for food. I've had the experience of being at the grocery store when I suddenly realize I'll never make it through the line and out to my car because I feel the fatigue overtaking me. I'll actually just leave all the groceries in the cart and go straight home to rest. It's better than collapsing there in the store! This is what I mean by knowing your limitations. The better you know yourself, and the more flexible you are willing to be, then, in the long run, the more goals you will accomplish."

Amye Leong is a remarkable woman, whose story is both inspirational and instructional. She offers us insight not only into the process of goal setting and attainment—key points in your arthritis game plan—but also into the workings and motivations of the human mind and psyche. If you would like further information on Young at Heart, contact:

11 Coral Tree Lane
Palos Verdes, CA 90274
213/377-2266

CHAPTER

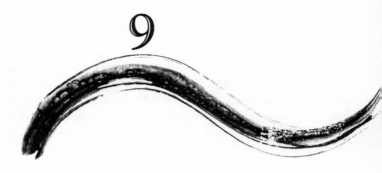

9

Failure:
The Key to Success

"Half the failures in life arise from pulling in one's horse
as he is leaping."

—A. W. HARE, *GUESSES AT TRUTH, I,* 1827

When Laura Kath was three years old she began
to experience pain in her feet and ankles. By age four the
pain had begun to spread upward. At age five she was diagnosed with rheumatoid arthritis. Her parents were told she
would never be a "normal" child because of the "disease."
Twenty-five years following that diagnosis, Laura Kath is still
involved with arthritis. But does she *have* arthritis? Was she
misdiagnosed as a child? Yes and no. Laura explains: "I was
diagnosed with arthritis at age five. I am currently *involved*
with arthritis. But I don't *have* arthritis. It isn't something I
want to own. I own a car, and I am glad that I own it. I own a

company, and I'm happy about that. But who wants to own arthritis?"

A unique way, indeed, of dealing with arthritis. But then, Laura Kath is a unique individual. Her story illustrates the general arthritis program principles discussed thus far, as well as demonstrating the particular principles I want to discuss in this chapter: turning failure into success, and arthritis into a learning, growing experience.

First I will discuss the concept of failure and redefine it in a way that success can be built out of failure. Then I will discuss some basic principles of how to turn failures into successes, and finally come back to Laura's story to see how this extraordinary and dynamic woman has turned a disease diagnosis into a prognosis of happiness and self-fulfillment.

A NEW DEFINITION OF FAILURE

It may seem odd that *Failure* (with an intended capital *F*) is here being presented as a key to success. After all, failure is usually defined as something that prevents success. In fact, my dictionary defines failure as a "a lack of success," "a deficiency," and "a falling short." Plus, the word "failure' has taken on a very pejorative sense in our culture. It doesn't just mean "falling short." It has come to imply that you are less of a person if you fail.

How in the world, then, can failure be redefined as a key to success? Yet that is precisely what it is in my motivational program. In fact, on at least one level this chapter is the anchor point of the entire book. If you can't learn to deal with *Failure*, then the rest of the superstructure will crack and eventually crumble. To carry this to what may seem like absurd lengths, failure is the most important thing any of us can do to ensure our success and happiness. In my program then, *Failure* is redefined as a learning experience in the process of goal achievement. How?

Failures and Successes Go Hand in Hand

If you follow through with your plan of goal attainment, then in theory your daily goals will help you meet your weekly goals, and your weekly goals will help you reach your monthly goals. If the monthly goals are accomplished, then the yearly goals should fall into place. In the end, if the yearly goals go as planned, then one's dream goals should be fulfilled. It logically follows, however, that the further into the future that the goal is set, the greater probability that something will interfere with the realization of that goal—some unforseen circumstance. The more things you try, the more things you will encounter that you both can and cannot do. Success, in this sense, means trying a lot of things, at which some you will succeed and at which some you won't.

The First Failures

The failure aspect of arthritis is always present. In the beginning when you are first diagnosed and are hurting so much, you seem to be experiencing constant failure because you're in a maze of trying to figure out what makes the pain go away. The only way to find this out is by trying, and trying always has the risk of failure. For example, trying different doctors, medications, or diets may or may not lead to pain relief. Most likely, especially in the early stages of rehabilitation, trying these different means of pain relief will result in some successes and some failures. For example, the copper bracelet didn't work, but the anti-inflammatory drug did. Or one anti-inflammatory drug didn't work but another one did. Each of these trial-and-error experiments resulted in both successes and failures.

Fear and Failure

The fear of failure has to be one of the worst of all emotions. Fear is one of the strongest negative emotions we have, because fear involves bad things: What if I try something and it doesn't work? What's the worst thing that could happen? Most of us think that the worst is something really horrible, when in reality it probably isn't that bad. We have to get over this concept of fear.

I have to admit that I was more than just a little afraid when I was in the hospital and I couldn't even move. You have to confront fear and ask yourself what's the worst and what's the best that could happen. Remember that it is better to try and fail than always wonder what might have been had you tried. For example, an initial fear of many people I've met with arthritis, and one that I had, is either never being able to walk again, or walking in so much pain that it will make life difficult to just get around on your own. But you can't let that stop you from trying. Sometimes the fear of failure is greater than the experience of failure. I tried over and over and over to walk, failing time and time again. But I could tell each time that I was getting stronger, so I kept trying and failing until I got it right. Then, when I could walk, I was afraid I wouldn't run. I went through the same process until I mastered that again. When I could run, I was still afraid people would know I was arthritic and that I would be an outcast or labeled a "cripple." In order to get over this fear, and especially this fear of failure, I thought of all the good things that could happen to me, and of all the little successes, even though they were small compared to the failures. That kept me going. I was after the bigger prize down the road—being healthy and strong again—and this prize would far outweigh all the failures put together.

FAILURE PRINCIPLES

There are a number of basic principles to be considered in dealing with goal achievement and the inevitable failure that can and will occur. These seven principles show you how you can make the failures and frustrations of arthritis work for you. I will first present them as general principles with some specific examples, and then return to the Laura Kath story to see how one person succeeded in applying these principles in her own way.

Be Flexible

The more things you try, the more change you will bring in your life, and much of it will be unexpected. If you are not expecting change, it can take you by surprise and leave you frustrated in being unable to complete your goal structure exactly as planned. But Helen Keller once said that "life is either a daring adventure, or nothing." If you want your life to be an adventure (in whatever relative way is adventurous for you), then be prepared for the surprises that all adventures entail. Enjoy change. Relish progress. But remember that with change comes the greater chance of failure if you are not flexible enough to make adjustments to those changes.

It is in this sense that I look at arthritis as an adventurous journey—a journey into the unknown. From the moment of diagnosis to whatever level of recovery you can achieve, each step along the way is new. For instance, you've never had to walk, eat, shower, or drive as you do now with arthritis. Because of this you must be flexible in making adjustments and learning to cope.

For example, when I got arthritis I was challenged as I had never been previously. Before when I was injured I took some time off to rest, then immediately jumped right back into my exercise routine to recover. But arthritis made the circumstances different. At first I was unable to just slip right into a routine like I had before. It took months, even years, of experimenting to find what worked for me. For the first six months I was constantly trying out new medications and combinations of anti-inflammatory drugs. Some didn't work at all. Others worked, but had terrible side effects. Still others worked with no bad side effects, but they prevented me from exercising at the level I wanted. Eventually I found the right combination and dosage for my body and needs.

But even with this example, flexibility is still the watchword, because my needs are still changing, even after all these years. I still experiment with different dosages, and this can vary from month to month, and from year to year. Don't forget that arthritis is a nonstatic, constantly-changing disease. It cycles you through highs and lows, and may even go into total remission for a time. So you've got to always be prepared for change.

Plus, your goals will constantly change as your body changes, so your goal plans must be flexible ones. As I'm sure you already know, arthritis makes each day a challenge, but the goal of this principle is to turn that challenge into an adventure by being flexible.

Take Calculated Risks

You should take risks, but you should not take them just as you please. There are timid risks, foolish risks, and the kind of risks I'm talking about—calculated risks. Somewhere there lies a balance between being too timid and not accomplishing what you are capable of, and being too bold and risking health or injury. That middle ground is the calculated risk.

Any level of goal achievement requires some amount of risk—without that it wouldn't be worth achieving. For example, one of the biggest risks I had to take at the beginning was simply learning to walk again. Trying to walk was a nonstop exercise in risk-taking and failure. I kept falling down. I couldn't get away from the crutches. But each time I tried to walk and fell, I learned not to do it that way again. With every fall I would get up knowing there was one less way I had to try. In this sense, the more I failed (fell) the closer I came to succeeding (walking) by narrowing down the possibility of choices. Each failure brought me closer to the right choice.

I dealt with this process with patience. I kept reassuring myself that I would walk again. I repeated over and over to myself, "It is going to happen again," and eventually it did. But it is important to remember that it didn't happen as fast as I wanted it to. But I never let go of the thought that it would happen. Finally it did, and those failures along the way became challenges to success.

For an arthritic, even something as basic as learning to walk again is quite a challenge and risk. But because the chances of failure may be raised to such a high degree, success becomes that much more valuable. In this sense, the fear of risks and failure can push you to higher expectations than you ever thought possible.

Don't Worry What Others Might Think

Everyone enjoys being recognized for his or her achievements. But with that comes the fear of what those same people will say or think if we fail, or if our goals seem too outlandish or farfetched. The thing about trying to succeed is that you will occasionally fail and others may criticize you. There is no magic solution to this problem. It's true—people do talk about other people they know (and even love). That too is part of human nature. The same people who applaud you for your successes may behind your back observe and maybe even relish your failures. All you can do is ignore these critics and go about your business. People will think what they will and there is nothing you can do about it. If you structured your life so that no one would think any negative thoughts about you, it would probably be a fairly boring life. The point is anyone can be a critic, so don't worry about what others might think. After all, it's the person who gets out there and tries who deserves the credit:

> It is not the critic who counts, not the man who points out how the strong man stumbled, or where the doer of deeds could have done them better. The credit belongs to the man who is actually

in the arena; who strives valiantly; who errs and comes short again and again; who knows great enthusiasm, the great devotions, and spends himself in a worthy cause; who at the best knows in the end the triumph of high achievement, and who at the worst, if he fails, at least fails while daring.

—Theodore Roosevelt

Failure Makes Success Appreciated

The possibility of great failure is what makes the triumph so sweet. Just as a valley creates an adjacent mountain, failure (or at least its possibility) makes fortune appreciated. According to Victor Frankel, the founder of logotherapy (a form of psychotherapy), people are not determined, but *self-determined.* "Man is both the sculptor and the marble," says Frankel. Logotherapy is an attempt to put the individual back in control of his life. Frankel believes that one of the key elements to finding meaning in life is to experience a certain amount of suffering. By suffering Frankel does not just mean pain. The doing of a deed and the experiencing of a value (two other elements in Frankel's formula for happiness) take on greater meaning when the deed or value is not easily had. I never realized what an accomplishment it is to be able to run or ride a bike until I suffered in trying to do so when I got arthritis. So many things I took for granted before are now daily triumphs. Arthritis has given me the chance to really appreciate everything I do. I will never again undervalue the simple things in life.

Every arthritis sufferer knows what it is like to wake up in the morning and have it be a struggle just to get out of bed and into the shower; a chore just to fix a meal, get dressed, and drive to work; a pain to work with your hands, lift objects, and walk or move quickly. All of these may be seen as forms of failure, but they may also be opportunities for appreciating the days when you get up and feel good, or even great; the days when you can jump out of bed, run to the shower, do your exercises and stretches and not hurt; the times when you can go about your day without suffering, and maybe even forget you have arthritis for a while. In this way failure can make success appreciated.

Let Your Lowest Moments Be Your Finest Hour

You should not only avoid seeing failures as low points, but embrace them as possibilities for great fortune. The next time you face a low motivation day, or a period when success at any level is seemingly unattainable, think of it as a golden moment to really prove yourself in the face of such adversity. In this sense, on the days when you awake feeling great, it is no real triumph to get up and do your chores, go to work, or finish a project. Of course, you celebrate this great feeling by doing just these things. But the glorification of self really comes when you *don't* wake up feeling great. The days when you are in pain are the very days that can be viewed as opportunities to prove yourself. Even if you can't do the things you could if you were not in pain, doing whatever you can is still a triumph because of the circumstances. No one, of course, would wish for these kinds of days, but when they come, look at them in this more positive way.

To keep his people motivated during the darkest days of the Battle of Britain in 1940, Winston Churchill effectively told them to see this not as an occasion for a weakening of the will, but as an opportunity for greatness:

> Do not let us speak of darker days; let us rather speak of sterner days. These are not dark days: these are great days—the greatest days our country has ever lived; and we must all thank God that we have been allowed, each of us according to our stations, to play a part in making these days memorable in the history of our race. Let us therefore brace ourselves that if the British Empire and its Commonwealth last for a thousand years men will still say, "This was their finest hour."

The More Chances of Failure
the More Chances of Success

There is one sure way to avoid failure altogether—not to try at all. This also ensures no success. For example, if you don't try to walk you sure as heck will never run again. It's possible that your arthritis is bad enough that running is out of the question, but if you don't try, then for sure it is out of the question! The point is that you just have to keep trying (and occasionally failing) until it all comes together. The more chances you take, the more chances you create for success.

In the beginning I was willing to try almost anything to relieve my arthritis. In fact, I did try almost everything. Most of what I tried didn't work. But I learned a lot on the way that I would not have had I not tried these various things. It's like trying different medications. The more you try, the more chances you create for finding the ones that work.

To use another example from sports, it is a fact that the greatest home run hitters in the history of baseball also tended to be the greatest strikeout kings. They were willing to take the risk of failing by swinging for the fences. Harold Helfer points out that "Babe Ruth's record of 714 home runs will never be forgotten. But how many of us know that the Babe struck out 1,330 times, a record rarely approached by any other player in the history of baseball." Think about each thing you try to improve yourself with as a time at bat—every medication, every diet combination, every exercise program, every doctor, every suggestion someone gives you. You never know which of these will be the home run.

Failures Are Learning Experiences

Finally, we should all look at failures as learning experiences, not defeating experiences. I've carefully kept track of all the different things I've tried in my experience with arthritis. This lets me look back and see what mistakes I've made, what worked and what didn't. You might even try keeping a personal journal, a diary of sorts, in which you make daily, weekly, or monthly entries on how you are feeling, your medication, your diet, your exercise program, your pain level, and so on. In this way you can look back and see any trends that might have developed, or any causal connections between something you tried and how you felt the following days or weeks.

For example, let's say for two months you changed medications to a new anti-inflammatory drug. In your journal you would note this, and then record any changes in how you feel on subsequent days and weeks over the next two months. At the end of that period you can look back to see how your body responded. You might even rank the level of pain on a scale of 1–10. Then you'll have an actual log of how you felt over that period of time. Then, let's say you switch medications for another two months, recording the changes in how you felt from day to day. At the end of it all, you can go back to the journal and draw some sound conclusions based on these simple experiments on yourself.

Thomas Edison "failed" over 6,000 times before he discovered that a carbonized cardboard filament would stay lit inside a glass globe for 170 hours—and in the process gave the world the electric light bulb. Another one of Edison's greatest achievements, the portable storage battery for automobiles, could also be judged as one of his greatest failures. Edison tried over 50,000 experimental models of storage batteries until he eventually hit upon the right combination of materials. Edison, in fact, kept track of his failures by cataloging them in large notebooks. In this manner he could look back to see what had been tried so that he would not have to try it again. On this level, then, we can look at Thomas Edison as one of the greatest failures in the history of technology. If there is anyone who could comment intelligently on the discovery of one's capabilities, it is Thomas Edison. After racking up an incredible 1,093 patents Edison said: "If we all did the things we are capable of doing, we would literally astound ourselves."

"THROUGH PAIN COMES POWER": THE LAURA KATH STORY

To put these principles into action means redefining failures as learning experiences you gain in the process of goal achievement. Laura Kath's life, in this sense, has been one long learning process. From the time of her diagnosis to the present she has built a full, rich, and successful life and career centered around the accomplishment of her goals by redefining not only failure, but arthritis and disease themselves.

Currently living in Santa Barbara, Laura is the founder of Young Adults With Arthritis (YAWA), vice-president of the Santa Barbara branch of the Arthritis Foundation, head of the Medical and Education Committee for the Arthritis Foundation, and camp counselor for Camp Esperanza, a juvenile arthritis camp in Big Bear, California. In her "spare time" she is owner and management consultant of Mariah Marketing, a company she founded several years ago. To keep her body in shape, both in general and to deal with the symptoms of arthritis, she stretches, does strengthening exercises, walks, bicycles, and sails.

This record of activities and accomplishments is obviously of someone who has redefined the limits of arthritis. Make no mistake about it, Laura Kath has had a full-blown case of rheumatoid arthritis all her life. From the time of her diagnosis at age five, she has suffered numerous setbacks that forced her to face the cruelties of life and the deep questions of meaning long before most. At the age of 13, a critical stage of development both physically and psychologically, Laura was forced to undergo synovectomies on both knees. "Basically the doctor told me I had two options," she recalled. "I could get the surgery or never walk again. Imagine a 13-year-old girl faced with a decision like that?!"

The decision was a major one indeed. At that time arthroscopic techniques had yet to be developed. Both of Laura's operations, separate for each knee, entailed a three-week stay in the hospital, followed by over two months on crutches, and another two years of physical therapy. "I realized at age 13 that there was no one else but myself who was going to make my life whole again. Only I could get myself out of the wheelchair and back on my feet. Most people don't have to face these kinds of decisions until later in life. Some people never have to face them. I decided as a young teenager what I wanted to do in life and when I wanted to do it."

For Laura that decision meant redefining arthritis and disease. "It's an issue of destiny. Who is in charge of yours? We are all owners of our lives, unless you decide to turn it over to someone or something else, like your doctor or arthritis. I was diagnosed with arthritis, but I don't have it. I am involved with arthritis, but it is not involved with me. I manage arthritis, it doesn't manage me."

This is the process of redefining. Laura Kath has turned failures into successes, and like everyone else, she certainly has had her share. "Oh, I get tired of taking the medication, or I don't feel like doing my stretching exercises, or I don't go for my walk or bicycle ride to keep loose, and then I pay for it later in pain." But Laura then turns these *failures* around. How does she do it? "I first examine the cause of the failure. I ask myself what was going on in my life when I failed and the pain came back. When you do this you generally discover what happened: you pushed yourself too hard, or you didn't rest enough, or you didn't take precautionary measures to protect your joints, or whatever." At this point Laura then makes a decision: "What do I want to do about this problem? Do I want to try to change the situation and learn from my mistake, or do I want to continue to suffer? For me, even if it is something I can't change, I at least change my attitude toward it."

Attitude is the key to Laura's methodology in dealing with her involvement with arthritis, and that attitude is summarized in one key phrase: "Through pain comes power." In this sense, Laura uses pain as a tool to drive herself and change her attitude. "My philosophy is that you can't change someone else's opinion, or some outside situation, but you can change your reaction to it. If you believe you are crippled, you *are* crippled. If you believe you are handicapped, you *are* handicapped. If you believe you have arthritis, you *have* arthritis. I simply choose not to believe that."

From this "pain is power" philosophy comes Laura's drive to share with others her unique philosophy. "This is why I've been involved with the Arthritis Foundation. I want to share with others these strategies I've developed. They may work for some but not for others. The point for me is to try. This is precisely why I've chosen to go public with my arthritis. The very process of discussing how I deal with my involvement with the disease has itself been a healing process. To get up and talk to an audience of a hundred people and tell them about your pain, that's what I mean by power!"

Laura also works toward public awareness of arthritis in young people. She wants to dispel the myth that arthritis only affects old people, and that if someone young has it they must be some kind of freak. Through public awareness, Laura hopes, will come support for the arthritis sufferer. "Having a strong support group is critically important. Your family and friends especially, but also groups you can go to and talk with others who share similar experiences as you, can help you realize that you are not alone, not abandoned." The degree of involvement, Laura says, is not as important as the process itself. "Just going to these meetings and listening to others discuss their involvement with arthritis is good enough for some people. You don't have to go and speak up or anything."

Support groups help build confidence in the arthritis patient through the power of positive attitude.

It sounds corny to talk about the "power of positive thinking" but the simple fact is, it works. Let me give you an example. When I was 18 years old I applied to attend Michigan State University to earn a degree in hotel management. When I told my doctor that I had been accepted, his first reaction was to offer to help me apply for handicap status. Maybe I could get a special parking place? Maybe I could get extra money? Maybe I could receive special services and favors? I remember I was startled at his comments. My jaw dropped. I had never really considered myself a handicapped person and here was my doctor not only putting that label on me, but suggesting I put the label on my car and everywhere else! Fortunately I was old enough and had been dealing with the disease long enough to ignore his suggestions. But even the idea irked me so that I remember it to this day. And as I look back at my treatment program I can see how he treated me as a handicap. This is what I mean by negative thinking.

The future for Laura Kath looks bright, as she continues to speak, write, and work with people who have been diagnosed with the same disease. "When I was 13 there was no one to turn to that understood what I was going through. I don't want that to be the case today. Now we have these support groups and I'm doing what I can to promote them."

INTELLIGENT FAILING

Our limitations and failures, then, are opportunities for taking new chances and winning new worlds. Failure is a necessary part of the arthritis challenge and the motivation program you design to deal with it. In fact, Jay Snelson, the director of the Institute for Human Progress, says that "failure is the *sine qua non* of success." Translated, this means that failure is an indispensable part of success. You simply cannot have one without the other. Snelson calls attention to Charles Kettering, a giant in the history of the automotive industry and the co-founder of the Sloan–Kettering center for cancer research, who once noted that "we must learn to fail intelligently, for failing is one of the greatest arts in the world." By this he meant that we learn from our failures and rise to higher levels of success because of them.

In this sense, having arthritis can be one tremendous learning experience for you. Though you may be confronted with pain and frustration and failure throughout your life, this pain can present problems you never encountered before. These problems and failures, in turn can be turned into opportunities for accomplishments. As Jay Snelson says, "the man who fails the least, accomplishes the least. The greater your ability to fail, the greater your achievement."

CHAPTER

10

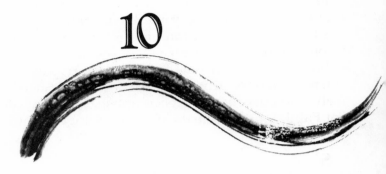

Destroying the Box: Integrating the Physical and Mental Challenge

"Imagination is the beginning of creation. You imagine what you desire; you will what you imagine; and at last you create what you will."

—George Bernard Shaw

As we have seen thus far, the challenges of arthritis, both physical and mental, are the stimuli to propel us to greater heights. Challenges are opportunities for us to test our physical and mental strengths and endurance. Arthritis is certainly not a challenge for which any of us asked, and if we could dispel these challenges I'm sure every single person out there would do so unhesitatingly. But we can't, so we've got to make the best of it. In this final chapter I want to integrate the physical and mental arthritis challenge concepts by discussing the relationship between body and mind. Not only does the body affect thoughts, but thoughts affect the body. The key to this linkage is creating thoughts that influence your body in the most positive way—that is, creatively restructuring your limitations to your advantage— what Frank Lloyd Wright calls "destroying the box."

DESTROYING THE BOX

We usually think of limitations as undesirable, yet we are in constant contact with them in every aspect of our lives. For the arthritis sufferer the simplest of tasks, such as opening doors or fixing a meal, can take on proportions of pain and frustration that the nonsufferer wouldn't understand. The key is to use these limitations as stimuli for creative and imaginative drives to greater heights and new frontiers, as the famed 20th-century architect Frank Lloyd Wright did in his architectural philosophy of "destroying the box." In such innovative designs as the Fallingwater house in the Allegheny mountains near Pittsburgh, and the Guggenheim Museum in New York City, Wright destroyed the confining concept of a building as a box, and became the stimulus for a century of creative growth in architecture. In fact, limitations triggered this burst of originality, as Wright *re-created* his constraints: "The human race built most nobly when limitations were greatest and, therefore, when most was required of imagination in order to build at all. Limitations seem to have always been the best friends of architecture."

To redefine your limitations you must first understand them and then consider how to work around them. For example, Martha Cooley's experiences illustrate this principle nicely. Her hands were too weak and inflamed to open doors, so she imaginatively learned to open them with her feet. She has creatively restructured her home (destroyed the box) to accommodate the new architecture of her body. It's not that her home is designed for a so-called "handicap," but that the arthritis challenge has stimulated her to new heights of creativity in her life. The point is that you can design an architecture around the limiting box of the new restrictions that have been put on you. Imagination and creativity are the keys to this new architecture.

Imagination and Creativity

Creativity will help you redefine your new limitations into a new architecture of success. To redefine your limitations, however, you have to understand them well enough to push beyond them. You must know the rules in order to break them, but not be so committed to these same rules that you can't visualize a new way around them. That's why it is important to understand the traditional limitations that physicians and arthritis experts offer, but not be so rigid as to believe that they must all apply to you. It is both good and important to read everything you can get your hands on about arthritis, and talk to the experts about the disease, but process this information as you need it, and then use it to break out of the traditional molds. This is a very fine line, and few ever make the transition from understanding the limitations to pushing beyond them. It takes both knowledge and imagination. For example, had I read and believed the Arthritis Foundation's advice about exercise and arthritis, namely that "exercise does not mean the kind pursued by an active, athletic person, such as vigorous sports or strenuous training sessions," I would never have completed any of my goals. Some arthritis sufferers can exercise like "an active, athletic person," and some can't. But the only way to find out is by trying. In Wright's metaphor, you should learn enough about the architecture of your body in order to be able to restructure it the way that best suits you.

Knowledge and Creativity

For most of us a lot of knowledge and intelligence actually stifles creativity. Psychology professor Robert Rosenthal of Harvard University did a fascinating study with people of exceptional intelligence and discovered a strong relationship between high I.Q. and the ability to successfully defend a point of view or idea. This, of course, makes sense. On the flip side, however, Rosenthal also found a strong relationship between high I.Q. and the inability to consider other alternatives. What happens is that more intelligent people are better able to convince themselves of the validity of a position, and defend it against attack from others, but are thereby committing themselves deeper to that stand. When a new or different way of viewing the problem arises, these intelligent people are less able to see it or accept it as tenable.

Thus your doctor, who is intelligent and strongly committed to the knowledge of arthritis he learned in medical school, is less likely to understand how to "destroy the box" than you are. This is why it is so important for you to take charge of your arthritic condition so that while you learn from your rheumatologist and therapist, you don't also let them define your limits. I can't emphasize enough that every case of arthritis is unique. You may have a certain type of arthritis that resembles someone else's, but how your body specifically deals with it and what your limitations are depend entirely on your specific case. Listen to authorities but don't accept any limitations unless you've discovered them yourself.

The difficulty in reconciling knowledge and creativity is never more obvious than in the health and medical fields. There is a constant battle between the old guard with their tried and true methods, and the new professionals with the latest techniques. Among the more conservative health experts, doctors, and therapists, there is an accepted dogma on what to eat, what drugs to try, which therapy is best, and so on. The balance between knowledge and imagination, however, is a delicate one. One doesn't want to be so open-minded that every new idea is embraced without careful thought and consideration regarding its validity. Believe me, I've tried everything imaginable to "cure" my arthritis, most of which was useless. Unfortunately there aren't any "miracle cures."

On the other hand, one doesn't want to be "stuck in the mud" and miss the excitement that new opportunities bring. It's a balance that must be carefully weighed by each individual in every unique situation. Carl Sagan explained this balance in an address to the Committee for the Scientific Investigation of Claims of the Paranormal (CSICOP), a group of scientists and medical doctors who investigate such health claims as cures for arthritis:

> What is so clearly called for is an exquisite balance between two conflicting needs—the most skeptical scrutiny of all hypotheses that are served up to us, and at the same time a great openness to new ideas. Clearly those two fight each other. But if you have only one of these you're in deep trouble. If you are only skeptical, then no new ideas make it through to you. You never learn anything new. But every now and then, maybe one in a hundred new ideas turns out to have wonderful, valid components to it and if you're too much in the habit of being skeptical of everything you're going to miss that. On the other hand, if you are open to every new idea and have not an ounce of skeptical sense in you then you cannot determine the useful ideas from the erroneous ones. If all ideas have equal validity then you are lost.

Redefine Your Limitations

The development of creativity and imagination has not escaped the scrutiny of psychologists. A typical test of creativity may be seen in the figure below. The instructions are to connect all nine dots with four consecutively drawn straight lines, without lifting the pen off the page. Try it on the figure.

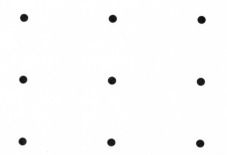

The solution, of course, is that you may draw the straight lines beyond the imaginary border created by the dots themselves. The border is imaginary because the instructions never said anything about staying within the borders. This is a literal example of "destroying the box." (The solution is presented at the end of the chapter.)

Such a limitation on thinking is what one must go beyond in creativity to solve the problem. In dealing with the limitations your arthritis puts on you, there are no pat answers to be found in any books on arthritis. There may be lots of suggestions on dealing with the problem, such as designing your home to be "arthritic friendly" (larger handles on utensils, well-lubricated drawers, doors for easy access, for example), but since your arthritis is unique to you, you must experiment for yourself to see what works.

THE PIGEONHOLE EFFECT

Imagination is the creative side of our thinking. We all think thoughts about ourselves. We all have a self-image. Much of that self-image is shaped and molded in our childhood and youth by parents, teachers, peers, and so on. But much of that self-image also comes from within, and there is no evidence that it cannot change. In fact, there is ample evidence that self-esteem can be greatly improved through techniques of visualization (see below). If we can apply creative imagination to games and sports, why not apply it to our self-esteem? We've got to think *something* about ourselves. Why not think something positive? This process is what Robert Rosenthal calls the "pigeonhole effect."

In 1965 Rosenthal and his colleague Lenore Jacobson conducted an experiment in an elementary school where children were given I.Q. tests at the beginning of the year. In 18 different classes the top 25 percent of the I.Q. scores were given to the teachers who were told that these kids were intellectual bloomers who would likely show marked improvement in their academic performance throughout the year. In actuality, Rosenthal and Jacobson had randomly assigned these scores, but by the end of the year these randomly chosen "bloomers" had indeed bloomed to the top of their class. Their grades had improved, and, more remarkably, so had their I.Q.s (which are supposed to be indications of ability, not achievement). Nearly half of them showed an increase of more than 20 points on the I.Q. test, a very significant difference.

Rosenthal and Jacobson explain these startling results as the pigeonhole effect—that is, expectation is a powerful motivator. The teachers expected more from the pupils labeled as bloomers, and therefore spent more time with them. Plus, these expectations were likely conveyed to the children, who then labeled themselves as bloomers, with a corresponding increase in their performance.

The point is that pigeonholing, labeling, and expectation all contribute to changing our image, both to others and ourselves. So why not pigeonhole yourself as a bloomer? Why not label yourself as a success? Why shouldn't you expect the most out of yourself? If you do, then you will, and so will others, with the likely result that you *will* be more successful. There is also evidence that such thinking can literally save your life.

THE THOUGHTS—HEALTH CONNECTION

We've seen how positive labeling and pigeonholing can influence your self-esteem and performance. Is it also possible that your thoughts can affect your health? There is evidence to support such a claim. In an article recently published in the *Journal of Personality and Social Psychology*, Christopher Peterson of the University of Michigan and Martin E. P. Seligman of the University of Pennsylvania reported the results of a study on the relationship between optimism or pessimism in attitude, and future health. In a 35-year longitudinal study, 99 Harvard University graduates were examined and questioned about their wartime experiences. They were asked about difficult personal situations encountered and how successfully the men felt they had handled them. They were also asked how the situations were related to work or health, and what physical or mental symptoms were experienced. The researchers then rated the explanations for optimism and pessimism. Dr. George E. Vaillant, a professor of psychiatry at Dartmouth Medical School, compared the medical data on the 99 men with data from extensive physical exams done every five years from age 25 to 60. Serious and chronic illnesses included heart disease, hypertension, and diabetes.

The results showed that those who offered pessimistic explanations at age 25 experienced more illness between ages 45 to 60 than the optimists. "I'm convinced," said Peterson, "there's a link between this personality characteristic and subsequent physical well-being." It is interesting that the effect is noticed in middle age, not youth. Perhaps herein lies the explanation for the relationship. It's not that an optimistic attitude has some magical effect on the body which prevents disease. It's that an optimistic attitude establishes a lifestyle which is conducive to health. Perhaps the pessimistic personalities neglect basic health care in the first place because they don't see life quite as worth living as the optimists. Once they become sick, maybe they fail to get help or follow medical advice. Seligman and Peterson reported that pessimists are often poor problem solvers and tend toward feelings of helplessness in situations. They feel that this might possibly lead to immune system suppression.

Scientists do not have a firm grip on the connection beween mental states and physical well-being. The field of *psycho-neuro-immunology*—the study of how our thoughts affect our nervous system, and how this in turn changes the immune system—is in an infant stage of development. We are only just beginning to understand that there is a link and that it is worth exploring. There are many different procedures for developing a working relationship between the mind and body. Each psychologist or sports trainer will have his own unique method. There is one, however, that is common throughout the field of psychology and therapy—visualization.

VISUALIZATION

Visualization is the process of focusing your thoughts and imagination on one thing. It is a process we all use. We all visualize things, whether we call it visualization or not. When we daydream, we are visualizing. When we just think about something, it is usually a picture we imagine. That is visualization.

Visualization is an important component of your program in taking up the challenge of arthritis. Visualization is a reaffirmation of what your goals are. It puts that extra stamp of approval on your goals. You aren't just thinking about it, you are seeing it happen—initially in your mind, later in life. I picture myself there and being successful, in whatever it is I'm doing—that's visualization.

Visualization is often subconscious. We do it anyway, so the trick is making what happens naturally—sometimes positive, sometimes negative—come out all positive. Since you are going to visualize anyway, why not do it in a manner that sets you up for success? I try to categorize my visualization according to the range of my goals. Visualizing is really just focusing on your goals.

For several years at the beginning of his cycling career Michael worked with a hypnotherapist who not only hypnotized him, but taught him visualization techniques so that he would no longer need her attending skills. He did this in order to gain control over pain and fatigue typically experienced in ultra-marathon cycling. Her methodology consisted of a three-part process that you can try right now, to visualize whatever you would like.

Part 1: The Tension–Relaxation Connection

In this step the individual is taught to understand what tension feels like in its extreme form, and then what it feels like to eliminate it. The purpose is to learn self-mastery and control over your body so that certain trained thoughts can control bodily functions. In this way you may learn to ignore pain, or at least control your reaction to it so that you can go about your normal activities with minimum interference.

1. Position yourself in a big easy chair or couch and feel relaxed and comfortable.

2. Squeeze your fist as tightly as possible for 15 seconds. Feel it shaking and note that the knuckles are white.

3. Relax your fist's grip and feel the tension flowing out of your arm and hand and into the air. As you note this feeling of relaxation, say to yourself in a slow easy fashion, "relax . . . relax . . . relax . . . ," over and over, until the association is made between the word "relax" and the feeling of tension relief.

4. Repeat steps 2 and 3 over and over again until the association is a strong one.

Part 2: Mastering Relaxation Throughout Your Body

In this part you will teach your entire body the relaxation process so that no matter where you are hurting you will learn to concentrate on that particular place to try to control the pain or tension:

1. Practice the process described in part 1, only do so for all the major sets of muscles in the body.

2. Begin with the toes. Clinch them up against the balls of your feet, hold for 15 seconds, relax, and repeat to yourself in the same manner as before, "relax . . . relax . . . relax," with the same associations.

3. Then move up to your ankles, calves, thighs, stomach, back, arms, shoulders, neck, and finally facial muscles. Repeat step 2 with each of the muscle groups until complete control over your body's muscular system is felt.

Part 3: Visualization

In part 3 the system established in parts 1 and 2 are applied to a particular situation:

1. Visualize yourself in a situation that is anxiety-producing. This can be anything that makes you feel tense or anxious, such as some task that causes pain and stiffness. An example might be doing a chore that is painful, yet must be done—like vacuuming, cleaning house, or going to the store for grocery shopping.

2. As you slip into that tension and anxiety, immediately say to yourself, "relax . . . relax . . . relax." If you have been practicing parts 1 and 2 then the tension and anxiety should decrease.

3. Repeat this sequence over and over until you feel you have mastery over your fears and anxieties.

4. Now, mentally place yourself in that situation that is anxiety-producing and repeat the above steps. See yourself vacuuming the carpet or going to the store. On the positive side, with this feeling of mastery and control over your mind and body, you can visualize yourself doing anything on your goal list, and "see" your success in that task. Go back to your list of goals and visualize yourself succeeding in them. Whatever it is, from the daily goals to the dream goal, imagine yourself making it, picture yourself doing it successfully. In this manner you can build your self-esteem and confidence.

In psychology this is known as progressive relaxation, systematic desensitization, or guided imagery, and is commonly used in therapy for phobias and anxiety attacks, as well as assertiveness training and confidence building. It is based upon the principle of incompatibility—the pairing of imaginary anxiety-producing scenes with the genuine state of physical relaxation. Because anxiety and relaxation are incompatible states, anxiety responses decrease as relaxation responses increase. These pairings are made in a hierarchical order, beginning with the least anxiety-producing scene and gradually progressing until the terminal scene, the most difficult situation, can be imagined without any feeling of anxiety.

These guidelines are rather general. What you specifically visualize will be unique to your situation. The point is to take something that bothers you—a limitation—and address it directly. What is it that makes it limiting and what can you do about it to change that situation? Let your imagination freely consider those possibilities, then try them out for real.

Sometimes these new ideas will work and sometimes they won't. But if you don't try anything, negative results are guaranteed.

Certainly visualization is not the only key to overcoming psychological problems in one's performance, but it is a useful technique that anyone can learn. While working with a therapist is ideal, it can be practiced from this simple three-part program.

THE VISUALIZATION—ARTHRITIS CONNECTION

For Martha Cooley, visualization is a key component in her program to deal with stress and her arthritis. Managing a household, family, and full-time job, in conjunction with having a fairly advanced case of osteoarthritis, gives Martha a sizable dose of stress all too often, for which she calls upon some techniques of visualization to handle. "Handling pain mentally means, for me, focusing on something other than the pain. When I practice visualization I will, for instance, think of something pleasant to distract my mind away from the pain."

For example, several years ago Martha took a class from a licensed hypnotherapist who trained her in making her own cassette tapes to listen to in times of stress and pain. "For me it was like listening to my own subconscious. The tapes have soft music playing in the background, over which comes your voice, or on some tapes I have the hypnotherapist's voice, telling me to relax, focus on another place, or another object other than the pain and stress. All I can tell you is that it works for me."

Focusing on colors is another technique Martha has developed. "Colors are hard to concentrate on for long periods of time, so when I am really stressed out and my arthritis is bothering me, I will sit down, close my eyes, and picture a color, say blue, and just concentrate on it, think about it, until

I forget about the pain." Martha has also used the toes-to-head relaxation technique described above (the Jacobson technique, as she learned it), and found it to be an effective way to get to sleep at night when her pain is bothering her. "If I can't fall asleep, I get up, fix a cup of something warm to drink, then lay back down and practice visualization until I fall asleep. If you keep trying, it eventually works."

An example of how positive visualization completely eliminated symptoms in a man diagnosed with rheumatoid arthritis is the case of Albert Kreinheder, a psychoanalyist who turned his therapeutic skills on himself and directly confronted his arthritis in a most unusual way:

Two years ago my life seemed to be flowing along beautifully. I had gained some respect in my profession, my health was excellent, and all in all I thought I was doing quiet well. At this seemingly high point in my life's achievements I was afflicted with rheumatoid arthritis. I had severe pain in every joint of my body, including even my jaw bones. After being awake for two or three hours and doing my normal sedentary activities, I would be exhausted and need to go back to bed. My shoulders and elbows were so stiff that unassisted, I couldn't put on my jacket nor without help could I rise from a prone position.

I tried everything, including physicians, chiropractors, nutritionists, masseuses, and tarot cards, but nothing seemed to work. Not knowing what else to do, I decided to talk to my pain. Here is a sample of the dialogues that materialized:

ME: You hold me tight in your grip, and you do not let me go. If you crave my undivided attention, you have received it. Whatever I attend to, I must also attend to you. Even when I write, I feel you in my hand, and always in all parts of my body. I am terribly frightened by you. I have no control over you, no access to you, no power to influence you. You need only go a little further, and then I am utterly helpless. Will you ever stop? Why are you here?

PAIN: I am here to get your attention. I make known my presence. I show you my power. I have a power beyond your power. My will surpasses yours. You cannot prevail over me, but I can easily prevail over you.

ME: But why must you destroy me with your power?

PAIN: I do so because I will no longer let you disregard me. You will bow down before me and humble yourself, for I am He of whom there is no other. I am the first of all things, and all things spring from me, and without me there is nothing. I want to be with you closely in your thoughts at all times. That is why I press you in the grip of my power and make you think only of me. Now, with my presence in yours, you can no longer live the same way and do the same things.

These dialogues gave meaning to my disability. Before, my pain was only a curse to be eliminated. Now it is revealed to be "He-of-whom-there-is-no-other." And this great-one desired intimacy with me. I became aware that my life had to change. When people are in the twenties, thirties, and perhaps through the forties, it is amazing to discover how totally ego-centered people can be and still prosper. But sooner or later, the larger personality asserts itself. "The time is coming," my pain said to me, "when I will put a stop to all those things that come before your love for me."

When a neurosis or a sickness comes to one, it does not mean that he is an inferior person with a defective character. In a way, it is a positive sign showing potentials for growth, as if within there is a greater personality pressing to the surface.

As bizarre as this process may seem, it worked for Dr. Kreinheder. In a recent seven-year follow-up it was reported that he is still completely symptom-free. While your approach to your pain need not take the form of a dialogue, the point is to confront it head-on. Take the problem by the scruff of the neck and *do* something about it. Use your pain, use your arthritis as a stimulus for growth. Your arthritic pain is an opportunity to release greater potential that you never knew was inside you.

VISUALIZATION SUGGESTIONS

The following is a list of some visualization scenes and thoughts on which you might try focusing whenever you feel especially stressed out or in excessive pain. After you've relaxed using the above techniques, visualize yourself in one of these special places, and then focus on these thoughts. By no means should you confine yourself to this list. This is just a starting point. Don't be shy about creating your own.

Places:

THE BEACH.   Visualize yourself lying on the soft, warm sand of a beautiful beach, with a gentle breeze cooling your face as the warm sun energizes your skin and body. Waves are rhythmically rolling in on the sand, creating a sensation of peace and tranquility in your mind and body. The clean ocean water cleanses the beach, just like your thoughts cleanse your body.

THE MOUNTAINS.   Visualize yourself sitting atop a grand mountain peak, safely perched on a large boulder overlooking the valley below. The sky is deep blue, the grass and trees are a rich green, and a wind whips through the valley below, echoing the sounds of nature that fall upon your ears like the gentle voices of the gods of nature. You feel good as you inhale the clean, cool mountain air. As you exhale you expel all tension, all pain, and you feel more and more relaxed with every breath. You haven't a worry in the world because you are on top of it.

BY A LAKE.   Visualize yourself far, far away, next to a beautiful, dark blue lake, surrounded by a rich forest of pine trees nestled atop gentle rolling hills, outlined by the clear blue sky. The wind sweeps across the lake, splashing the water onto the shore, while little birds skirt along the lake edge. The sun is warm in your face, and warms your body, making all your joints feel loose and supple, and all pain is gone because in this special place, pain is not allowed. Joy and happiness, feelings of warmth, both physical and mental, overcome your body so that you can feel nothing but pleasure.

BY A STREAM. Visualize yourself far up a valley surrounded by sharp, jagged mountains, whose high peaks protect you from the hot sun beyond, and create a wonderful wind that sweeps down the valley and washes over your face, causing the blood to rush to your skin and making you feel flush with joy in being at one with nature. You've hiked a long way along the path of the stream, and now you've found a comfortable place on some small rounded pebbles next to the stream. The water flows down the stream, carrying with it any and all impurities, just like your blood flows through your body, carrying with it anything that doesn't belong. In this place you haven't a worry in the world. Nothing matters outside of this valley. It is just you and the natural creation. No stress, no worries, no responsibilities, and especially no pain. This is the valley of peace and the stream of life.

Thoughts:

PHYSICALLY AND MENTALLY RELAXED.   In your special place focus on the fact that your body and your mind are completely relaxed. You have no worries, no stress, and especially no pain, so there is no reason why you shouldn't be relaxed. As you repeat the words "relax," "relaax," "relaaax," you are becoming more and more comfortable in your place. Tension, stress, and pain flow out of your body, never to return. You feel good because you are relaxed. And when you are relaxed, you can't feel anything but good.

SELF-CONTROL.   Now that you are relaxed, you are in control. It is your body. It is your mind. In your special place you have achieved self-mastery and self-control. Nothing can take that away from you, and even when you return from your special place you will remain in control. No disease, no body, no thing can take that control away from you because it is yours. You own self-control. And once you own it, it is yours forever. You will never let it go.

OPTIMISTIC AND CONFIDENT.   Now that you are in control, you feel optimistic and confident. Optimism and confidence are things that you can choose to have. Since you control your body, your thoughts alone can make you feel confident. You feel good about yourself. You are a worthy person, as worthy as anyone else alive. There is no one who can make such judgments about you, so why not make them yourself? You can do almost anything, if you are confident enough. And since you are in control of your body, you can certainly will it to feel good. Make your body feel good now. It is your body. You control it. Command it to feel good, and know that your positive outlook will make it happen.

HIGH ENERGY.   Now that you feel optimistic and confident about your body, your mind, and the world around you, you will suddenly come across new forms of energy you've never encountered. Your body swells with energy. With each breath you take, your lungs transmit that energy throughout your body. With each heartbeat your blood carries the energy brought in by your lungs to the rest of your body. From your toes to your head you feel charged—supercharged, in fact. This energy will enable you to overcome any obstacle, any pain, any conflict in your life. There is nothing you can't do, because this energy will drive you forward.

THE MIND–BODY CONNECTION

Such visualization techniques work, not because of magic, but because of the mind–body connection. Recent research into how the mind and body interact reveals that these are not two separate elements, but two manifestations of the same element. The philosophical split between mind and body, initiated by the French philosopher René Descartes in the 18th century, is now being mended. Mind and body are two sides of the same coin, and understanding this may not only improve your arthritic symptoms and overall health, it may literally save your life.

The case and life story of Norman Cousins has now become a fountainhead of a new generation's challenge to traditional medical models of healing, and bears repeating here, as among the many physical ailments Cousins suffered in 1979 was ankylosing spondylitis, the same form of rheumatoid arthritis with which I've been diagnosed. Cousins's two books, his classic *Anatomy of an Illness* and his more recent *The Healing Heart*, illustrate the mind–body connection in a powerful way. At the age of 10 Cousins was diagnosed as having tuberculosis and was sent to a sanitarium for six months where he received a real-world education on the importance of a positive mental attitude:

> What was most interesting to me about that early experience was that patients divided themselves into two groups: those who were confident they would beat back the disease and be able to resume normal lives, and those who resigned themselves to a prolonged and even fatal illness. Those of us who held to the optimistic view became good friends, involved ourselves in creative activities, and had little to do with the patients who had resigned themselves to the worst. When newcomers arrived at the hospital, we did our best to recruit them before the bleak brigade went to work.
>
> I couldn't help being impressed with the fact that the boys in my group had a far higher percentage of "discharged as cured" outcomes than the kids in the other group. Even at the age of ten, I was being philosophically conditioned; I became aware of the power of the mind in overcoming disease. The lessons I learned about hope at that time played an important part in my complete recovery and in the feeling I have had since about the preciousness of life.

Cousins, now adjunct professor at UCLA's School of Medicine, was diagnosed as having an arthritic and rheumatoid-like collagen disease of the connective tissues—ankylosing spondylitis. In a well-documented recovery program he treated himself with large doses of positive mental attitude and good humor, mainly in the form of Marx Brothers movies and "Candid Camera" reruns. Sound ridiculous? Maybe. But it can work. In fact, his more recent recovery from a heart attack was documented and analyzed by four heart specialists who concluded the following factors were instrumental in the mind–body connection with Cousins:

1. The absence of panic in the face of the obviously grave symptoms of his heart attack.

2. His unshakable confidence in his body's ability to utilize its own wisdom in facilitating healing.

3. An irrepressible good humor and cheerfulness that created an auspicious, healing environment for himself, as well as for the entire hospital staff.

4. Taking a full share of responsibility for his recovery by establishing a close "partner relationship" with his physicians.

5. His focus on creativity and meaningful goals, which made recovery worth fighting for and life worth living.

Creating a New Physical and Mental Architecture

The Arthritis Foundation is correct in its warnings about nonscientific claims of arthritic cures and treatments. We don't want to make any claims here that somehow positive thoughts and visualization are going to magically improve your arthritis symptoms. There is much experimental evidence, however, in support of the effectiveness of the method in altering your perception of reality. For example, in an experiment with children in a gymnastics skill imagery task, one group physically practiced on the horizontal bars five minutes a day for six straight days. Another group physically practiced on the bars for the same duration, but were also given a guided imagery task in which a gymnastics instructor took them through a five-minute practice session on the horizontal bars. A third control-group did neither. Later, all the children were tested in a horizontal bars skills task and rated by gymnastics instructors on their abilities. As might be expected, those who actually physically practiced did better than those who did nothing, but not surprisingly, and to the point, those who did both the physical practice *and* the guided imagery fared the best. It's true. Seeing yourself succeed *does* help you become successful.

Such experimental and scientific evidence for the power of imagination and creativity in helping us overcome or redefine our limitations is encouraging. This imagery is nothing special. Whenever you daydream or just let your mind wander (or wonder), you are practicing visualization and imagery. Since your thoughts affect your body, why not think positively, why not create a new physical and mental architecture for yourself?

In dealing with your arthritis imagine yourself successfully completing some task that has become difficult for you to do because of your arthritis. I do this every morning when I get up. I imagine myself getting around the house, doing my daily chores, driving down to the pool, swimming my laps, driving to work and doing my job successfully, going for a bike ride or run after work, and so on. Such visualizations keep up the positive mental attitude that you are not going to let arthritis keep you down.

Integrating Mind and Body

Integrating the physical and mental challenge of arthritis means making the mind–body connection. For example, in a list of diseases for which the "placebo effect" works in producing at least 50 percent relief, rheumatoid arthritis is one of them. In effect, arthritic patients given placebos ("sugar pills" or inactive substances), not knowing whether they were being given real pain killers or the placebo, received at least 50 percent pain reduction!

In spite of much skepticism within the medical fellowship, there is now substantial evidence within the psychological community of the connection between personality, emotion, and illness. In the early 1900s there was a heavy bias for an organic explanation of disease. In the late 1950s and early 1960s much research was conducted that gave credence to the idea that the mind can and does affect the body. Psychosomatic disorders were discovered, in which it became clear that it was the mind causing the actual physiological problems. Physical disorders such as migraine headaches, asthma, hypertension, ulcers, and circulatory impairments often occur in the absence of known organic causes. In these cases the organic dysfunction or damage is believed to be directly related to psychological components.

To achieve a state of wellness (if only relative to certain unalterable physical conditions) clearly we need an approach different from the one we were raised to believe would make us whole. This integration of physical activity with psychological and social dynamics, can and does lead to more confidence in all facets of life.

It is becoming clear that the mind can and does affect the body. Psychosomatic disorders are potent reminders of the negative power of the mind. Author and holistic physician Jack Schwarz, who teaches a course entitled Voluntary Controls of Internal States, once related a story about a woman who came to him with an allergy for roses. Later Jack put roses on the table before her and she immediately experienced an allergic reaction. Then, as a demonstration of the power of the mind, he informed her that the roses were replicas, not the real thing! Such placebo effects are well documented in the psychological literature.

The courses offered by Schwarz teach the principles of the powers of the mind through meditation. Jack shows how one can learn to voluntarily control such bodily functions as sleep, pulse rate, blood pressure, pain, fatigue, and even bleeding. As an unusual example of extreme control, Jack eats one meal a day and sleeps two hours a night. He can control his bleeding, immunize himself to infection, and feel no pain when a large carpet needle is thrust through his arm (as personally witnessed by Michael). According to Dr. Elmer Green of the Menninger Foundation (a highly respected research institute in the field of experimental psychology), Jack Schwarz "has, in the realm of voluntary controls, one of the greatest talents in the country and probably the world."

In a reversal of a common term in psychology, Schwarz stresses that if there can be psychosomatic effects, then there can also be somatopsychic effects. In other words, it's a two-way street. Not only does the mind affect the body, but the body can affect the mind. Depending on the physical condition of the body, the mind can feel good or bad.

Since I've gotten arthritis and have been meeting others who have the disease, I am struck by the number of people who let this disease beat them down. The pain really depresses them, so they sit around and think of how miserable they feel, which makes the pain even worse because they are concentrating on it. This makes them even more depressed, which, in turn, makes the pain even worse, and so on. They get caught in this vicious cycle and they can't get out.

So what do you do if you are in that negative cycle? Reverse your thinking. Think positive thoughts. Practice the visualization techniques, picturing yourself symptom-free, successful, happy, and healthy, and bouncing around your environment. Think of how positive you feel about yourself when your body is in good physical condition. The condition of the mind parallels the condition of the body. If you don't feel good physically, it is evident in all words and actions. When you feel good you have more energy. Mind and body cannot be separated. They go hand in hand. The ascent of one means the escalation of the other. The downfall of one means the collapse of the other. The balance and integration of mind and body will lead to a greater level of wellness— and thus happiness—making whatever your condition a more pleasant one in which to be.

REMOVING YOUR REINS

In the movie *Equus,* based on the play by Peter Shaffer, the psychiatrist Dr. Martin Dysart (played by Richard Burton) has the job of "curing" the adolescent Alan Strang, whose passionate obsession with horses has led him to commit the heinous deed of gouging out the eyes of several of the beasts he loves so much. Dysart discovers the deep-seated psychological link between the boy's passion and his crime, but in the process learns that it is he himself who may be in need of "curing." Strang is in emotional pain, but he is wild, passionate, and carefree. Dysart has no emotional pain, but he is conservative, staid, and cautious. Strang has gone to the extremes with his love, albeit for a mythological beast. Dysart, in his prudency, has lost all hope of ever loving again: "That boy has known a passion more ferocious than I have known in any second in my life, and I envy it." And to Strang, at the successful end of therapy, Dysart tells him: "Passion can be destroyed by a doctor. It cannot be created. You won't gallop any more, Alan." But in the end it is the doctor who realizes the incurable paradox of the necessity of risking pain in order to have passion; of knowing your limitations in order to transcend them:

> You see, I'm lost. I wearing that horse's head myself, all reined up in old language and old assumptions, straining to jump clean hooved onto a whole new tract of being I only suspect is there. I can't see it because my educated average head is being held at the wrong angle. I can't jump because the bit forbids it and my horse power is too little. There is in my mouth this chomp chain, and it never comes out.

As Frank Lloyd Wright pointed out in his "destroying the box" metaphor, it is limitations that define what we should and should not do, but not necssarily what we *can* and *cannot* do. In order to experience highs, they must be defined by lows. Peaks, in part, are created by valleys, and valleys by peaks. Only with the risk of the worst can come the best. Only with the risk of foolishness can come wisdom. Only with the risk of despair can come hope. Only with the risk of having nothing can come everything.

The puzzle solution to breaking out of the box:

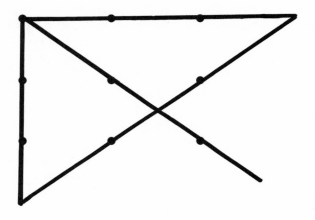

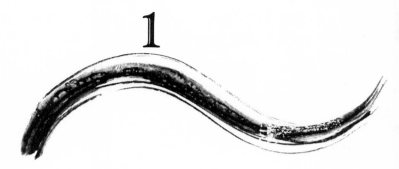

Arthritis Foundation Chapters

One of the first things you should do when you take up the physical and mental challenges of arthritis is to contact your local chapter of the Arthritis Foundation. They can supply you with additional information about the disease, doctors, and therapists in your area who have worked with the Arthritis Foundation, as well as support groups that meet regularly to discuss the many aspects of both the physical and mental challenge of arthritis.

One of the important elements of my motivational program is to get reinforcement and feedback from others who have also been diagnosed with arthritis. From them you can learn new strategies in dealing with the disease, different ways of coping, new drugs or exercises, or means of doing things around the house or job that make it easier on your joints. The Arthritis Foundation organizes many social and public activities to raise funds for research in treatment and cures, which are also great ways to get involved and take the problem by the scruff of the neck so that you feel like you are doing something constructive toward the betterment of your life and the lives of others like you.

NATIONAL HEADQUARTERS:

The Arthritis Foundation
1314 Spring St., N.W.
Atlanta, GA 30309
(404) 872-7100

BY STATE:

ALABAMA

Alabama Chapter
17 Office Park Circle
Birmingham, AL 35223
(205) 870-4700

South Alabama Chapter
1720 Springhill Avenue
Mobile, AL 36604
(205) 432-7171

ALASKA

Alaska Unit
c/o Western Area Office
2422 Arden Way, Suite A-28
Sacramento, CA 95825
(916) 924-1878

ARIZONA

Central Arizona Chapter
711 East Missouri Avenue
Suite 116
Phoenix, AZ 85014
(602) 264-7679

Southern Arizona Chapter
4500 East Grant Road
Tucson, AZ 85712
(602) 326-2811

ARKANSAS

Arkansas Chapter
6213 Lee Avenue
Little Rock, AR 72205
(501) 664-7242

CALIFORNIA

Northeastern California Chapter
2422 Arden Way
Suite A-28
Sacramento, CA 95825
(916) 921-5533

Northern California Chapter
203 Willow Street
Suite 201
San Francisco, CA 94109
(415) 673-6882

San Diego Chapter
7675 Dagget Street
Suite 330
San Diego, CA 92111-2241
(619) 492-1094

Southern California Chapter
4311 Wilshire Boulevard
Suite 530
Los Angeles, CA 90010
(213) 938-6111

COLORADO

Rocky Mountain Chapter
2280 South Albion Street
Denver, CO 80222
(303) 756-8622

CONNECTICUT

Connecticut Chapter
1092 Elm Street
Rocky Hill, CT 06067
(203) 563-1177

DELAWARE

Delaware Chapter
222 Philadelphia Pike, #1
Wilmington, DE 19809
(302) 764-8254

DISTRICT OF COLUMBIA

Metro Washington Chapter
1901 Ft. Myer Drive
Suite 500
Arlington, VA 22209
(703) 276-7555

FLORIDA

Florida Chapter
5211 Manatee Avenue, West
Bradenton, FL 34209
(813) 795-3010

GEORGIA

Georgia Chapter
2045 Peachtree Road, NE, #800
Atlanta, GA 30309-1405
(404) 351-0454

HAWAII

Hawaii Chapter
200 N. Vineyard Boulevard
Suite 503
Honolulu, HI 96817
(808) 523-7561

IDAHO

Idaho Chapter
4696 Overland Road
Suite 538
Boise, ID 83705
(208) 344-7102

ILLINOIS

Central Illinois Chapter
2621 N. Knoxville
Peoria, IL 61604
(309) 682-6600

Illinois Chapter
79 W. Monroe Street, Suite 510
Chicago, IL 60603
(312) 782-1367

INDIANA

Indiana Chapter
8646 Guion Road
Indianapolis, IN 46268
(317) 879-0321

IOWA

Iowa Chapter
8410 Hickman, Suite A
Des Moines, IA 50322
(515) 278-0636

KANSAS

Kansas Chapter
1602 East Waterman
Wichita, KS 67211
(316) 263-0116

KENTUCKY

Kentucky Chapter
3900 B. DuPont Square South
Louisville, KY 40207-4615
(502) 893-9771

LOUISIANA

Louisiana Chapter
3955 Government Street
Suite 7
Baton Rouge, LA 70806
(504) 387-6932

MAINE

Maine Chapter
37 Mill Street
Brunswick, ME 04011
(207) 729-4453

MARYLAND

Maryland Chapter
3 Lan Lea Drive
Lutherville, MD 21093
(301) 561-8090

MASSACHUSETTS

Massachusetts Chapter
450 Chatham Center
29 Crafts Street
Newton, MA 02160
(617) 244-1800

MICHIGAN

Michigan Chapter
23999 Northwestern Highway
Suite 210
Southfield, MI 48075
(313) 350-3030

MINNESOTA

Minnesota Chapter
122 W. Franklin
Suite 215
Minneapolis, MN 55404
(612) 874-1201

MISSISSIPPI

Mississippi Chapter
6055 Ridgewood Road
Jackson, MS 39211
(601) 956-3371

MISSOURI

Eastern Missouri Chapter
7315 Manchester
St. Louis, MO 63143
(314) 644-3488

Western Missouri/
Greater Kansas City Chapter
8301 State Line
Suite 200
Kansas City, MO 64114
(816) 361-7002

MONTANA

Montana Chapter
1500 Poly Drive
Billings, MT 59102
(406) 248-7602

NEBRASKA

Nebraska Chapter
2229 North 91st Court
Suite 33
Omaha, NE 68134
(402) 391-8000

NEVADA

Nevada Chapter
3850 W. Desert Inn Road
#108
Las Vegas, NV 89102
(702) 367-1626

NEW HAMPSHIRE

New Hampshire Chapter
P.O. Box 369
35 Pleasant Street
Concord, NH 03302
(603) 224-9322

NEW JERSEY

New Jersey Chapter
200 Middlesex Turnpike
Iselin, NJ 08830
(201) 283-4300

NEW MEXICO

New Mexico Chapter
124 Alvarado, S.E.
P.O. Box 8022
Albuquerque, NM 87108
(505) 265-1545

NEW YORK

Central New York Chapter
The Pickard Building, Suite 123
5858 East Molloy Road
Syracuse, NY 13211
(315) 455-8553

Genessee Valley Chapter
One Mount Hope Road
Rochester, NY 14620-1088
(716) 423-9490

Long Island Chapter
501 Walt Whitman Road
Melville, NY 11747
(516) 427-8272

New York Chapter
67 Irving Place
New York, NY 10003
(212) 477-8310

Northeastern New York Chapter
1237 Central Avenue
Albany, NY 12205
(518) 459-5082

Western New York Chapter
1370 Niagara Falls Boulevard
Tonawanda, NY 14150
(716) 837-8600

NORTH CAROLINA

North Carolina Chapter
3801 Wake Forest Road
#115
Durham, NC 27703
(919) 596-3360

NORTH DAKOTA

Dakota Chapter
115 Roberts Street
Fargo, ND 58102
(701) 237-3310

OHIO

Central Ohio Chapter
2501 North Star Road
Columbus, OH 43221
(614) 488-0777

Northeastern Ohio Chapter
23811 Chagrin Boulevard
Chagrin Plaza East, Suite 210
Beachwood, OH 44122
(216) 831-7000

Northwestern Ohio Chapter
2650 North Reynolds Road
Toledo, OH 43615
(419) 537-0888

Southwestern Ohio Chapter
7811 Laurel Avenue
Cincinnati, OH 45243
(513) 271-4545

OKLAHOMA

Eastern Oklahoma Chapter
4520 W. Harvard, #100
Tulsa, OK 74135
(918) 743-4526

Oklahoma Chapter
2915 Classen Boulevard
#325
Oklahoma City, OK 73106
(405) 521-0066

OREGON

Oregon Chapter
4445 S.W. Barbur Boulevard
Portland, OR 97201
(503) 222-7246

PENNSYLVANIA

Central Pennsylvania Chapter
P.O. Box 668
2019 Chestnut Street
Camp Hill, PA 17011
(717) 763-0900

Eastern Pennsylvania Chapter
1217 Sansom Street
Philadelphia, PA 19107
(215) 574-9480

Western Pennsylvania Chapter
Warner Centre—Fifth Floor
332 Fifth Avenue
Pittsburgh, PA 15222
(412) 566-1645

RHODE ISLAND

Rhode Island Chapter
850 Waterman Avenue
East Providence, RI 02914
(401) 434-5792

SOUTH CAROLINA

South Carolina Chapter
1802 Sumter Street
Columbia, SC 29201
(803) 254-6702

TENNESSEE

Middle-East Tennessee Chapter
210 25th Avenue, North
#807
Nashville, TN 37203
(615) 329-3431

West Tennessee Chapter
6084 Apple Tree Drive
Suite 4
Memphis, TN 38115
(901) 365-7080

TEXAS

North Texas Chapter
2824 Swiss Avenue
Dallas, TX 75204
(214) 826-4361

Northwest Texas Chapter
3145 McCart Avenue
Fort Worth, TX 76110
(817) 926-7733

South Central Texas Chapter
1407 N. Main
San Antonio, TX 78212
(512) 224-8222

Texas Gulf Coast Chapter
7660 Wood Way
Suite 540
Houston, TX 77063
(713) 785-2360

UTAH

Utah Chapter
1733 South 1100 East
Salt Lake City, UT 84105
(801) 486-4993

VERMONT

**Vermont &
Northern New York Chapter**
P.O. Box 422
Burlington, VT 05402
(802) 864-4988

VIRGINIA

Virginia Chapter
565 Southlake Boulevard
Richmond, VA 23236
(804) 270-1229

WASHINGTON

Washington State Chapter
100 South King, #300
Seattle, WA 98104
(206) 622-1378

WEST VIRGINIA

West Virginia Chapter
P.O. Box 296
Dunbar, WV 25064
(304) 768-3667

WISCONSIN

Wisconsin Chapter
8556 West National Avenue
West Allis, WI 53227
(414) 321-3933

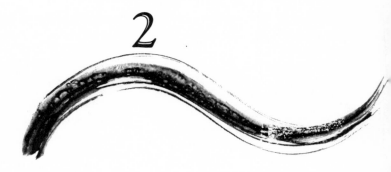

National Institute of Arthritis and Musculoskeletal and Skin Diseases (NIAMS) Centers

Certain medical research institutions throughout the United States have been selected to receive funds from the National Institute of Arthritis and Musculoskeletal and Skin Diseases (NIAMS). Difficult arthritic cases requiring complex treatments may be referred to one of these centers.

NEW ENGLAND

Boston University Arthritis Center
Evans Medical Group
80 East Concord St.
Boston, MA 02118
(617) 638-7460

Robert B. Brigham Arthritis Center
Brigham & Women's Hospital
75 Francis St.
Boston, MA 02115
(617) 732-5325

Division of Rheumatic Diseases,
University of Connecticut Health
Center
School of Medicine
Farmington, CT 06032
(203) 679-2160

MIDDLE ATLANTIC

The Rheumatic Disease Clinic at
the Hospital for Special Surgery
Cornell University
535 East 70th St.
New York, N.Y. 10021
(212) 606-1328

SOUTH

Duke University Arthritis Center
Clinic
Rheumatology Appointments
Coordinator
Box 3809
Durham, NC 27710
(919) 684-3956

UAB Arthritis Center
University of Alabama
Medical Center
Russell Ambulatory Center
1813 Sixth Ave. South
Birmingham, AL 35294
(205) 934-1443

University of North Carolina
Thurston Arthritis Research
Center
932 FLOB, Room 231H, CB#7280
Chapel Hill, NC 27599
(919) 966-4191

University of Tennessee
Department of Medicine
956 Court Ave., G326
Memphis, TN 38163
(901) 528-5737

The University of Texas
Southwestern Medical Center
at Dallas
Division of Rheumatic Diseases
5323 Harry Hines Blvd.
Dallas, TX 75235-9060

MIDWEST

Northwestern Medical Faculty
Foundation
222 East Superior St.
Chicago, IL 60611
(312) 908-8628

Special pediatric arthritis
division at:
Children's Memorial Hospital
2300 Children's Plaza
Chicago, IL 60614
(312) 880-4360

Indiana University Multipurpose
Arthritis Center
541 Clinical Dr.
Indianapolis, IN 46223
(317) 274-4225

Section of Rheumatology
Rush-Presbyterian–St. Luke's
Medical Center
1725 W. Harrison, Suite 1098
Chicago, IL 60612
(312) 942-8268

**University Hospitals Arthritis and
Spine Center at Case Western
Reserve University**
2074 Abington Rd.
Cleveland, OH 44106
(216) 844-3168

**University of Michigan Hospitals
Department of Internal Medicine
Division of Rheumatology**
3918 Taubman Ctr.
Ann Arbor, MI 48109-0352
(313) 936-5491

**Department of Orthopedic
Surgery
University of Minnesota**
420 Delaware St. SE
Box 189
Minneapolis, MN 55455
(612) 625-1177

PACIFIC

**Rosalind Russell Arthritis Center
University of California Medical
Center**
400 Parnassus Ave.
San Francisco, CA 94143
(415) 476-1192

**Scripps Clinic and Research
Foundation
Division of Rheumatology**
10666 North Torrey Pines Rd.
La Jolla, CA 92037
(619) 554-8585

**Stanford Immunology and
Rheumatology Clinic**
S-101 Stanford Medical Center
Stanford, CA 94305
(415) 723-6001

**University of California School of
Medicine
Department of Medicine
Professional Group,
Rheumatology**
UCLA-CHS 47-139
10833 Le Conte Ave.
Los Angeles, CA 90024-1736

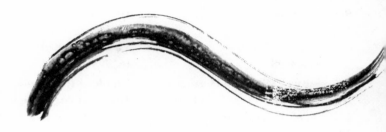

Bibliography

The following list of books was compiled for the purposes of directing the reader toward further information on arthritis, without attempting to offer recommendations or reviews. Arthritis Foundation publications are listed first, followed by other general and specific books about arthritis.

ARTHRITIS FOUNDATION PUBLICATIONS

All listings (unless noted otherwise) are brochures that can be obtained for free by writing the Arthritis Foundation at P.O. Box 19000, Atlanta, Georgia 30326. Brochure numbers are listed after the names of the brochures.

Arthritis and Employment. #9070.

Arthritis and Farmers. #9327.

Arthritis and Travel. #9071.

Arthritis Today (Bimonthly magazine available for a $15.00 or more membership contribution to the Arthritis Foundation.)

Basic Facts. #4001.

Coping and Pain. #9333.

Coping with Stress. #9326.

Diet. #4280.

Exercise and Your Arthritis. #9704.

The Family—Making the Difference. #9334.

Guide to Insurance for People with Arthritis. #9332.

Guide to Laboratory Tests. #9060.

Guide to Medications. #9059.

Guide to Social Security Disability Insurance for People with Arthritis. #2230.

Help Your Doctor—Help Yourself. #9325.

Living and Loving. #9190.

Overcoming Rheumatoid Arthritis (Spiral-bound book available for a fee.) #4083.

Practical Information. #4100.

Research: What's New. #4221.

Serious Look. #5785.

Surgery. #4230

Taking Care. #9329.

Taking Charge. #4221.

Understanding Arthritis. (Book). 1984. New York: Scribners.

Unproven Remedies. #4240.

We Can: A Home Care Guide for Parents of Children with Arthritis. (Spiral-bound book available at a fee.) #9749.

When Your Student Has Arthritis. #9560.

Types of Arthritis:

Ankylosing Spondylitis. #9050.
Arthritis and Inflammatory Bowel Disease. #9062.

Arthritis in Children. #4160.

Back Pain. #4370.

Behcet's Syndrome. #9065.

Bursitis, Tendinitis & Myofascial Pain. #9055.

Carpal Tunnel Syndrome. #9728.

Fibrositis. #4340.

Gout. #4180.

Infectious Arthritis. #4360.

Inherited Disorders of Connective Tissue. #9063.

Osteoarthritis. #4040.

Osteonecrosis. #9337.

Paget's Disease. #9064.

Polymyalgia Rheumatica. #4330.

Polymyositis/Dermatomyositis. #4390.

Pseudogout. #9054.

Psoriatic Arthritis. #9053.

Raynaud's Phenomenon. #9324.

Reflex Sympathetic Dystrophy Syndrome. #9061.

Reiter's Syndrome. #4350.

Rheumatoid Arthritis. #4020.

Sarcoidosis. #9057.

Scleroderma. #9051.

Sjögren's Syndrome. #9328.

Systemic Lupus Erythematosus. #9052.

The Vasculitides. #9056.

Medication Briefs:

Aspirin. #4260.

Azathioprine (Imuran). #9355.

Corticosteroids (Steroids). #9220.

Cyclophosphamide (Cytoxan). #9360.

Diflunisal (Dolobid). #9322.

Fenoprofen (Nalfon). #9120.

Gold. #4120.

Hydroxycholoroquine (Plaquenil). #9200.

Ibuprofen (Motrin, Rufen). #9140.

Indomethacin (Indocin). #9240.

Meclofenamate (Meclomen). #9340.

Methotrexate. #9350.

Naproxen (Naprosyn). #9180.

Penicillamine (Cuprimine, Depen). #9300.

Piroxicam (Feldene). #9321.

Sulindac (Clinoril). #9320.

Tolmetin (Tolectin). #9160.

General Bibliography

Bingham, Beverly. 1985. *Cooking with Fragile Hands: Kitchen Help for Arthritics.* Naples, Fl.: Creative Cuisine, Inc.

Bland, John. 1960. *Arthritis Medical Treatment and Home Care.* London: Collier Macmillan.

Blau, Sheldon, and Dodi Schultz. 1973. *Arthritis.* Garden City, N.Y.: Doubleday.

Calabro, John, and John Wykert. 1971. *The Truth About Arthritis Care.* New York: McKay.

Chamberlain, B. Charmaine. 1982. *Stop Arthritis Pain.* Alameda, Calif.: Ascot Group Publishers.

Ellert, Gwen. 1985. *Arthritis and Exercise: A User's Guide to Fitness and Independence.* Vancouver, B.C.: Trelle Enterprises, Inc.

Friedman, JoAnn. 1986. *Home Health Care—A Complete Guide for Parents and Health Professionals.* New York: W. W. Norton.

Fries, James. 1986. *Arthritis. The Comprehensive Guide to Understanding Your Arthritis.* New York: Addison-Wesley Publishing.

Gach, Michael. 1989. *Arthritis Relief at Your Fingertips.* New York: Warner Books.

Goldfarb, L., M. J. Brotherson, J. A. Summers, and A. P. Turnbull. 1986. *Meeting the Challenge of Disability or Chronic Illness: A Family Guide.* Baltimore: Paul Brooks Publishing Co.

Healey, Louis, Kenneth Wilske, and Bob Hansen. 1977. *Beyond the Copper Bracelet.* Bowie, Md.: Charles Press.

Jayson, Malcolm, and Alan St. J. Dixon. 1974. *Understanding Arthritis and Rheumatism.* New York: Dell.

Jayson, Malcolm, and Alan St. J. Dixon. 1980. *Rheumatism and Arthritis.* London: Pan Books, Ltd.

Jetter, Judy, and Nancy Kadlec. 1985. *The Arthritis Book of Water Exercises.* New York: Holt, Rinehart and Winston.

Jones, Monica Loose. 1985. *Home Care for the Chronically Ill or Disabled Child—A Manual and Sourcebook for Parents and Professionals.* New York: Harper and Row, Inc.

Keough, Carol. 1983. *Natural Relief for Arthritis.* Emmaus, Pa.: Rodale Press.

Lemaistre, JoAnn. 1985. *Beyond Rage—The Emotional Impact of Chronic Physical Illness.* Oak Park, Ill.: Alpine Guild.

Lewis, Kathleen. 1985. *Successful Living with Chronic Illness—Celebrate the Joys of Life.* Wayne, N.J.: Avery Publishing Group.

Lorig, Kate, and James Fries. 1986. *The Arthritis Helpbook: A Tested Self-Management Program for Coping with Your Arthritis.* New York: Addison-Wesley Publishing.

Mervyn, Leonard. 1986. *Rheumatism and Arthritis.* New York: Thornsons Publishing.

Moskowitz, Roland, and Marie Haug. *Arthritis and the Elderly.* New York: Springer Publishing Co.

Physician's Desk Reference (PDR). 1990. Oradell, N.J.: Medical Economics Co.

Pitzele, Sefra. 1985. *We Are Not Alone: Learning to Live with Chronic Illness.* Minneapolis, Minn.: Thompson and Co.

Portnow, Jay, and Martha Houtman. 1987. *Home Care for the Elderly—A Complete Guide.* New York: McGraw-Hill Book Co.

Rooney, Theodore, and Patty Rooney. 1985. *The Arthritis Handbook.* Dubuque, Iowa: William C. Brown, Inc.

Simonton, Carl. 1983. *Getting Well Again.* New York: Houghton Mifflin.

Stern, Edward. 1981. *Prescription Drugs and Their Side Effects.* New York: Grosset and Dunlap.

Wallace, Jean. 1989. *Arthritis Relief.* Emmaus, Pa.: Rodale Press.

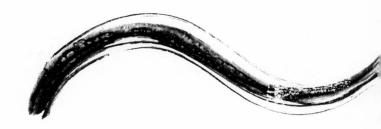

Index

ABOUT THE AUTHORS

GEORGE YATES is a 35-year-old professional triathlete, fitness consultant, and member of the Board of Governors for the Southern California Chapter of the Arthritis Foundation. The Laguna Beach, California resident was struck down by acute ankylosing spondylitis, a type of rheumatoid arthritis, in 1983. From complete immobilization to once again successfully competing in the Hawaiian Ironman Triathlon in October 1985, George's intense two-year program of exercise therapy and psychological preparation has set new standards in the arthritis field for the role of both the body and the mind in learning to live with arthritis. He tours the country giving motivational talks to arthritis groups and professional athletes alike, emphasizing the importance of a positive mental attitude in overcoming adversity.

MICHAEL BRANT SHERMER is Assistant Professor of Psychology at Glendale College, in Glendale, California, where he teaches courses in psychology, evolution, and the history of science. He has a bachelor's degree in psychology from Pepperdine University and a master's degree in experimental psychology from California State University, Fullerton. He is currently completing a doctorate in the history of science at Claremont Graduate School, publishes regularly in scholarly journals, and is author of *Teach Your Child Science*. Michael Shermer also races bicycles, having enjoyed a career as an endurance cyclist. He is one of the founders of and five-time participant in the Race Across America. He has several published books on cycling and sports psychology, including *Psychling, Sport Cycling, Cycling: Endurance and Speed, The Woman Cyclist,* and *The RAAM Book.*